Innate Defense: Cells & Function

Chris

Table of Contents

CHAPTER 1:
INTRODUCTION

1.1 Literature Review

1.1.1 The Immune system

The Immune system consists of cells, organs, tissues and protein that enables the body to fight against pathogens including viruses, bacteria, parasites and others including dead cells destined to be cleared by the system. The immune system is made of the innate and adaptive arms (Murphy 2011)

1.1.2 Innate Immunity

The Innate immunity is the first line of defence during the invasion by a pathogen, it was originally thought to be non-specific, but can distinguish between self and invading pathogens or non-self that potentially cause damage. The first line of the immune defence comprises of the skin, while inside the body mast cells, eosinophils, basophils, Natural killer cells are involved. Most importantly, phagocytic cells including macrophages, neutrophils and dendritic cells, identify and eliminate invading pathogens. Pattern-recognition receptors (PRRS) on the surface of cells, recognise components on microbes known as pathogen-associated molecular patterns (PAMPs). In *Mycobacterium tuberculosis*, the lipids and polysaccharides of the cell wall, are recognised mainly by Toll-like receptor 2(TLR2) and TLR4, which are also known to play a role towards the initiation of the adaptive immunity during *Mycobacterium tuberculosis* (*Mtb*) infection. Control *L monocytogenes*, on the other hand, depends on the activation and signalling through TLR2, though TLR5, TLR9 has been shown to also play an important role. Specific interaction of PRR and PAMPs leads to the activation of cascade signalling pathways leading to host-protective responses. This leads to the recruitment of other cells into the site of infection through the release of chemokines and cytokines. Macrophages are the major phagocytes in the immune system, there are various forms depending on their location and origin. Macrophages are distributed throughout the body, for example, we have alveolar macrophage which is resident on the lungs and established during embryonic development with tissue-specific function from a foetal liver origin and monocyte-derived macrophage which are differentiated into macrophages during inflammatory conditions. Depending on the pathogen/macrophage interaction, macrophages differentiate into two different subsets, classically activated macrophages or M1 macrophages, or alternatively activate macrophages or M2 macrophages. M1 macrophages are induced by Th1 cytokines interferon-gamma (IFN-γ), or by lipopolysaccharide (LPS). Uptake of the intracellular pathogen by macrophages results in the production of reactive nitrogen intermediates (RNIs) such as nitric oxide (NO) and reactive oxygen species (Gordon 2003). On the contrary, M2 macrophages induce arginase 1 production and decrease NO and have regulatory activities with wound healing functions (Figure 1.1) (Classen *et al.* 2009; Martinez *et al.* 2009), with a combination of IL-1β or LPS or IL-10, TGF-β producing cytokines contribute towards immune regulation balance.

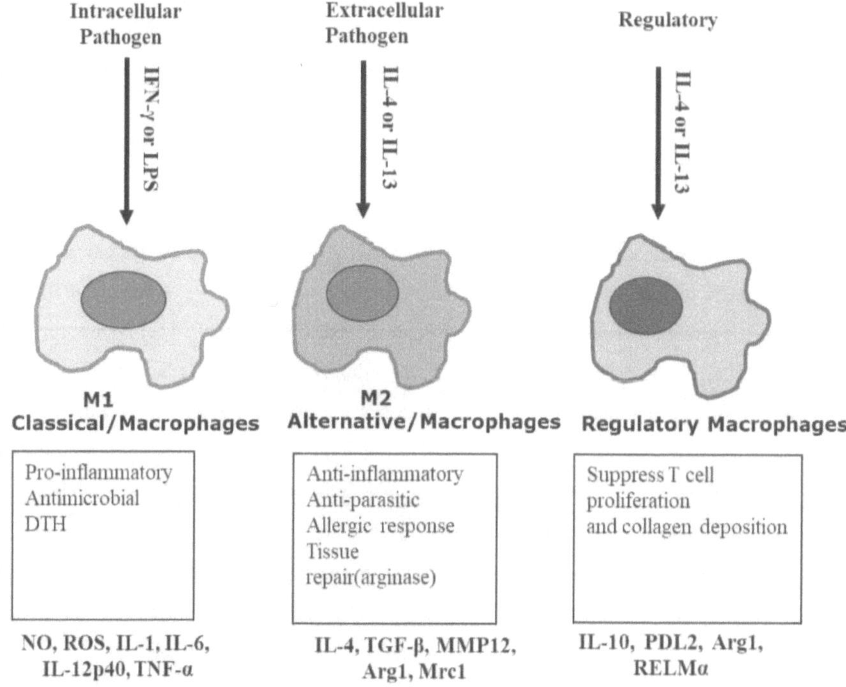

Figure 1. 1 Schematic illustration of Pathogen interaction with macrophages: Classical activation of macrophages (M1 macrophages induced) by Th1 cytokines in combination with stimuli (IFN-γ or GM-CSF) and/or with microbial components like lipopolysaccharide (LPS) induce a pro-inflammatory phenotype. M2 Macrophages (alternative) activated by Th2 cytokines (IL-4/IL-13). [Adapted and redrawn from (Gordon 2003; Murray & Wynn 2011)

Neutrophils or polymorphonuclear neutrophils (PMN) are the most abundant group of innate cells, they are also phagocytic cells, by engulfing and killing pathogens. Eosinophils release eosinophils protease, which plays an important role in tissue remodelling and the targeting of large parasites that cannot be phagocytosed. Natural Killer (NK) cells have the ability to kill tumour cells following the loss of MHC-I, they are known to produce IFN-γ and TNF-α which act on macrophages to enhance the immune response. Dendritic cells (DCs) are the major antigen-presenting cells (APCs) but also play a role in the degrading of evading pathogens. There are different types of DCs, and their location is associated with their function. However, their major role remains the linking of the innate immunity and the adaptive immunity, through their ability to take and process antigens and migrate to secondary lymphoid organs where they present to T cells to initiate the immune response (Medzhitov & Janeway 2000; Akira *et al.* 2006)

1.1.3 Adaptive Immunity

Activation of the adaptive immunity is orchestrated by the innate immune system when it does not successfully eradicate invading pathogen, initiation is typically delayed and but when activated, it mounts defences that are specific to the exposed antigens. There is immunological memory after exposure to a particular antigen. Adaptive immunity is base on two arms, the humoral and cell-mediated immunity. Infected antigen-presenting cells (APC) migrate to the lymph nodes to cross-talk with T cells leading to clonal expansion of antigen-specific T cells. At the lymph nodes, CD8$^+$ and CD4$^+$ T cells are activated via MHC-I and MHC-II antigen presentations respectively. γδ T-cells and NK T-cells also expand during activation and display immune effector functions. Adaptive immunity expresses a large repertoire of genetic recombination both in antibodies/immunoglobulins and T cell receptors allowing the recognition of a broad spectrum of pathogens and misformed or altered self cells.

CD8$^+$ T cells have been shown to protect intracellular pathogens like *Mtb* and *Lm* against intracellular pathogens. Mice lacking MHC-I have been shown to be susceptible to immune response to tuberculosis and listeriosis (Finelli *et al.* 1999; Sousa *et al.* 2000) with studies in humans having a similar effect (Cooper 2009; Bruns *et al.* 2009) CD8$^+$ T cells play an important role most especially against bacteria located in the cytoplasm like *Lm*. CD8$^+$ T cells directly kill infected cells by the release of granules like granzymes and perforin (Kaufmann

1993) these cells also indirectly assist in the killing of pathogens by the production of IFN-γ and TNF-α that recruits macrophages (Ngai *et al.* 2007).

CD4[+] T cells play a pivotal role in intracellular pathogens located inside the vacuole such as *Mtb*. The role of CD4[+] T cells in tuberculosis has been supported by the fact that HIV virus induces depletion CD4[+] T cells, which are essetial in maintaining latently infected tuberculosis patient. Depletion of CD4 T cells leads some of these patients developing active tuberculosis, hence the link between these diseases in co-infection settings (Geldmacher *et al.* 2012).

CD4[+] T cells polarise into different subsets, depending on the antigenic peptides and cytokines during infection. These subsets include Th1, Th2, ThFH, Th17 and T reg with an enhanced or protective outcome, depending on the immune response. Some of the subsets are discussed below.

Th1 cells are characterised by the presence of the transcription factors T-bet and Signal transducer and activator of transcription 4 (STAT4) which are required for their development (Szabo *et al.* 2000; Thieu *et al.* 2008). Th1 cells develop in response to viruses and intracellular pathogen which are essential for clearance. Activation is occastrated, by the secretion of IL-12 by macrophages which ochastrate the activation of CD4 T cells to produce IFN-γ. This antimicrobial activity is the central effector action of Th1 cells. IFN-γ activates macrophage antimicrobial effector pathways like inducible nitric oxide synthase (iNOS), upregulating the expression of ROIs and RNIs. IFN-γ also plays a major role for the maturation of phagosome, acidification, autophagy and Vitamin D receptor signalling (Chan *et al.* 1992; MacMicking *et al.* 2003; Gutierrez *et al.* 2004) Mice lacking INF-γ produced by CD4 T cells have been shown to susceptible to *Mtb* infection. Though other subsets such as NK cells, CD8[+] cells, CD1-restricted, γδ Tcells secrete IFN-γ, CD4[+]T cells remain the major source. The other subset cannot adequately compensate for the production of IFN-γ in the absence of CD4[+] cells. (O'Garra *et al.* 2013). Other cytokines critical for the control of intracellular pathogens are IL-12 and TNF. TNF like IFN-γ is crucial in both humans and mice for immunity to TB (Bean *et al.* 1999), patients on anti-TNF for rheumatic diseases have been shown to have a fivefold risk factor to develop active TB (Keane *et al.* 2001). Though production of such key cytokines by Th1 cells does not necessarily translate into protection against disease suggesting other key factors are required for the protective interplay. It is, for this reason, the central dogma of IFN-γ secretion is neccesarry but not sufficient for protection against Tuberculosis (Nunes-Alves *et al.* 2014).

Th2 cells are important for extracellular parasites, such as in asthma and allergic diseases. Similar to Th1 cells, Th2 differentiate from CD4$^+$ T cells. GATA3 and STAT6 are key transcription factors necessary for their differentiation and expression (Zhu 2010). Th2 cells release IL-4, IL-5, IL-13, and IL-10 cytokines that suppress or control immune response during phagocyte-independent responses. IL-4 receptor alpha chain (IL-4Rα)/STAT6/GATA3 and IL-2/STAT5 signalling through Th2 cell are vital for Th2 differentiation. Th2 play a role in intracellular diseases in damping inflammation or subverting immune killing. IL-4 and IL-13 have been shown to be upregulated in active Tuberculosis patients with a corresponding downregulation of Th1 responses (Seah *et al.* 2000; Harris *et al.* 2007). Antigen triggering producing key cytokine IL-4 plays a major role in the differentiation of CD4+ naïve T cells, and also neutralises macrophage antimicrobial activity by reversing the actions of IFN-γ, and GM-CSF (Bhattacharya *et al.* 2015).

Th17 T cells have as major transcription factor RORγt and STAT3 that are essential for the modulating and balancing of these cells. STAT3 is known to have a pleiotropic function and not specific to Th17 cells only, therefore RORγt remains the definding transcritptional factor (Durant *et al.* 2010). Th17 cells arise at the peripheral from the differentiation of CD4$^+$ Naïve T cells, induced by IL-23, IL-6 and TGF-β. Their secretion is associated with the defends against autoimmune disease, fungi and extracellular bacteria. (Durant *et al.* 2010) Th17 cells are also known to produce IFN-γ during active tuberculosis disease, but a shift in the production of IL-17 during the active state is known to recruit neutrophils which may be detrimental and causes tissue damage during active tuberculosis (Torrado & Cooper 2010).

T regulatory cells (Tregs) are another very important Th subset, they express the forkhead box P3 (Foxp3) helix as a transcriptional factor. Foxp3 determines the T cell lineage in addition to CD4,$^+$ CD25$^+$ under naïve state. CD25$^+$ is not a marker during infection this is so because effector T cells also express CD25$^+$ (IL-2Rα), making it difficult to distinguish Tregs without the crucial Foxp3 transcriptional factor. The ectopic expression of Foxp3 in other tissues or cellular poulation has been shown to perform similar regulatory functions therby confirming their expression signify T cell regulatotion (Hori *et al.* 2003). Mutation of Foxp3 in humans leads to the development of multiorgan autoimmune disease, allergy, and immune dysregulation, polyendocrinopathy X -linked (IPEX) syndrome (Zhu *et al.* 2017) There are two subsets of Tregs natural Tregs (nTregs), developing directly from the thymus and inducible Tregs (iTregs) which are induced from CD4$^+$ naïve cells at the periphery in response to an antigen, TGF-β and IL-2. (La Cava 2008). T regs play a major role to maintain immune tolerance to self-antigens by secreting the cytokines TGF-β, IL-10 which have an inhibitory effect in response to immune activation during infection. T regs also alter the activation and differentiation of antigen-presenting cells thereby delaying the differentiation of CD4$^+$ T cells during infection (Bluestone & Tang 2005).

Though Th1, Th2, Th17 and Tregs discussed above are the major lineages, there are more recent subsets like Follicular helper T cells (Tfh) expressing Bcl6 as its transcriptional factor that assist B cells in the production of antibodies (Hale & Ahmed 2015). Wide range of plasticity has been suggested in different T cells, suggesting differentiation is not terminal and subject to differences depending on the circumstances (O'Shea & Paul 2010). Plasticity of the tranditional linages are well known, with individual lineages that could produce signature cytokines of other subsets under certain condition, for example, IL-10 is produced by Th1, Th2, T regs and Th17 cells subsets, though normally secreted by T regs (Veldhoen *et al.* 2008; Saraiva *et al.* 2009). The understanding of class-switching during infection and the conditions influencing these differences are important for theurapuetic purposes. The different subsets can also express more than one transcriptional signature with different functions. T regs expressing both Foxp3 and RORγt (O'Shea & Paul 2010) under certain conditions, suggesting other factors like cellular differentiation, epigenetics can influence the function. Ex-Foxp3 cells have been known to acquire the capacity to produce predominantly Th1 cytokines like IFN-γ or IL-17 for Th17 cells (Xu *et al.* 2007; Wei *et al.* 2009; Zhu 2010), and also Th2 cytokines such as IL-4, IL-13 (Pelly *et al.* 2017).

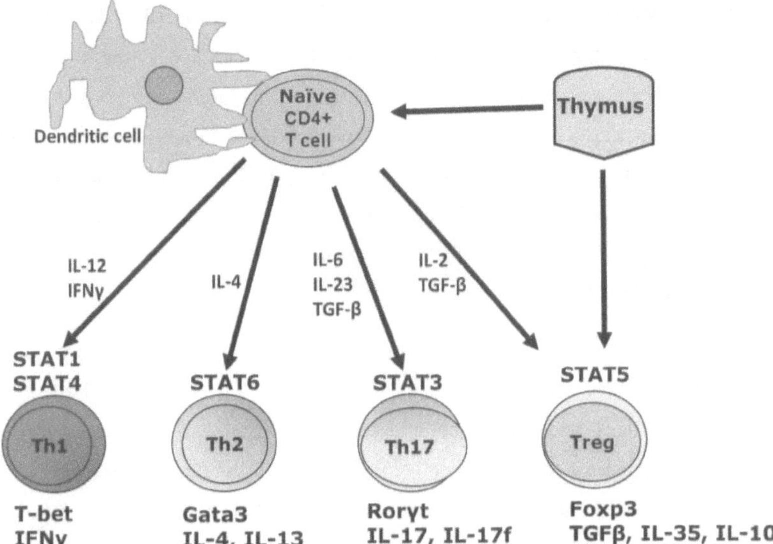

Figure 1. 2 T Helper cell differentiation according to traditional lineages Differentiation of CD4 T cells: Dendritic cell presenting MHC-II loaded antigen to naïve CD4[+] T cell, with their master transcriptional regulatory factor. These subsets produce certain cytokines as illustrated above but recent studies show this cytokine is not limited to fixed linages but there is growing evidence of plasticity among different subgroups depending on the pathogen condition. Image source from (O'Shea & Paul 2010).

Studies on the role of IL-4 on the effect of T regs have been inconclusive. Addition of IL-4 on Th2 cells was shown to reduce the effect of T regs suppression, similarly in another study treatment of Th2 T cells with monoclonal antibody anti-IL-4 led to the depleting of T regs. (Cosmi *et al.* 2004; Tu *et al.* 2017).In addition, exposure of IL-4 on Tregs prevented apoptosis and conserving Foxp3, leading to T reg survival and potency, translating into controlling naïve CD4[+] T cells (Pace *et al.* 2005; Maerten *et al.* 2005)

1.1.4 Cytokines

Cytokines are small proteins (low molecular weight) including chemokines, interferons, interleukins, lymphokines and tumour necrosis factors released by myeloid cells like neurophils, macrophages and dendretic cells, T cells CD4 and CD8 during immune activation play a vital for cell signalling. They have pleiotropic effects which include the regulation of innate and adaptive immune responses. Their release affects cells around them, leading to the recruitment of other cells including neutrophils and macrophages (Vilček & Feldmann 2004). Cytokines act in an autocrine manner, affecting the cells that secrete them, paracrine, affecting the surrounding cells, or endocrine manner affecting cells away from the area of secretion, however, they are very distinct from hormones. Cytokines play a primordial role in the differentiation, proliferation of immune cells. (Dempsey *et al.* 2003). Their responses are essential for host survival but are also detrimental in disease if not well controled or regulated. For example, IFN-γ is important for defence against intracellular pathogens like *Lm* and *Mtb* and most autoimmune diseases. Inadequate regulation or excessive secretion has been shown to cause tissue damage in viral and bacterial infections (Davidson *et al.* 2015). Also, IL-2 is required for cytotoxic T cells (CTL) generation also required for most vaccines, however, it drives graft/host disease and is involved in bone marrow transplantation. (Dinarello 2007)

There are currently thirty-three interleukins, with the IL-1 family with eleven members including IL-1α, IL-β, IL-18, and IL-33, having well-described overlapping functions within the family involved in pro-inflammatory secretion. The IL-6 family includes the IL-11, leukaemia inhibitory factor, oncostatin ciliary neurotropic factor and cardiotropin-1, members activate hepatic acute proteins. The IL-10 family has as member IL-22 which play an important role in damping or regulating inflammatory responses. IL-2, IL-7, IL-9, IL-15, IL-21 perform similar functions in promoting T cell differentiation into effector T cells and memory T cells during immune activation (Liao *et al.* 2011). The colony stimulation factors (CSF) such as granulocyte-CSF, granulocyte-macrophage CSF, have distinct genes and receptors but perform overlapping functions in promoting myeloid cell proliferation and maturation. There are several types of chemokines, classified into four main groups, they act as a chemoattractant in the migration of cells. There also act in homeostasis, angiogenesis and cellular maturation and wound healing.

Table 1. 1 Different types of cytokine their sources, and targeted cells with brief but not limited biological functions.

Factors	Source	Target cells	Biological activity
IL-1a, b	Monocytes, B Cells, Dendritic Cells, Macrophages	T and B Cells, Liver	Pyrogenic reaction, Lymphocyte activation, inflammatory mediator.
IL-2	T cells(Th0, TH1), NK Cells	T and B Cells, NK Cells	Activation, Proliferation of T and B Cells, Isotype switching
IL-4	Th2 Lymphocytes, B Cells , Macrophages	T and B cells, Macrophages	Activation, growth and differentiation
IL-5	T cells, Macrophages	Eosinophils, Lymphocytes	Chemotactic and activating factor for eosinophils and lymphocytes
IL-6	B and T Cells, Macrophages, Endothelium	Eosinophils, Lymphocytes	Proliferation, production of acute phase proteins. B cell differentiation factor
IL-7	Bone marrow, thermic, epithelium	T and B pro-lymphocytes or immature Cells	Lymphocyte cell growth factor
IL-8	Macrophages, Endothelium, T cells	Neutrophils, Eosinophils, T Cells	Neutrophils, T Cells, Chemotactic factor
IL-10	Macrophages, T and B Cells	Macrophages, Mast cells, T Cells	Growth factor regulator
IL-12	Monocytes, Macrophages, Neutrophils, Dendritic Cells B Cells	NK cells, T Cells, Macrophages	Activation of NK Cells, T cells,
IL-17	Activated T Cells	T Cells	Promotes T Cell proliferation
GM-CSF, G-CSF, M-CSF	Macrophages, T Cells, Mast Cells, NK Cells	Macrophages Dendritic cells	Promote inducible haematopoiesis
TNF-α	Macrophages , T Cells, NK Cells, Neutrophils, Mast cells Eosinophils	T cells , Macrophages	Regulate immune cells. Pyrogenic and induces apoptotic cell death

1.2 *Listeria monocytogenes*

Listeria monocytogenes (*Lm*) is a gram-positive facultative anaerobic rod-shaped (0.4 by 1-1.5μm) and are non-spore/capsule forming and no capsule, of low G+C content. It is the cause of listeriosis in humans and most mammals. It is a foodborne disease and broadly found in nature. The presence of *Lm* is found on ready to eat foods products (unpasteurized milk, cheeses, raw vegetable, ice cream, lunch meats and refrigerated smoked seafood). Infections occur when humans consume contaminated food products. *Lm* is highly tolerant to salt, and acidic conditions and can grow, survive at low temperatures. Tracking the source of is challenging, this is so because the time frame of infection and the incubation is long. It takes from 3 to over 70 days for illness to develop clinical symptoms which include fever, headache, muscle aches and non-specific syptoms like chills. Illness can be mild in immunocompetent individuals, but high risk individuals like children, pregnant women and the elderly, the infection can be lethal. (Ferreira *et al.* 2014). In certain cases, serious blood infection (septicemia) can occur (Figure 1.3), inflammation of the brain (encephalitis), inflammation of the spinal cord (miningitis). In mothers with *Lm* infection, outward symptoms may not appear, the fetus might be seriously affected. These individuals are unable to develop adapted and redrawn from (Sahibzada *et al.* 2017) adequate immune response to *Lm* infection. *Lm* grows in both phagocytic and non-phagocytic cells, easily handled in vitro and grows in tissue cultured cells. The immune system clears off the invasion in low doses in immunocompetent individuals, however, high doses consumption of food infested with *Lm*, results in gastrointestinal problems. In mouse models, infections and their dynamics are fast, which makes it an ideal pathogen to study both innate and adaptive immunity for intracellular pathogens.

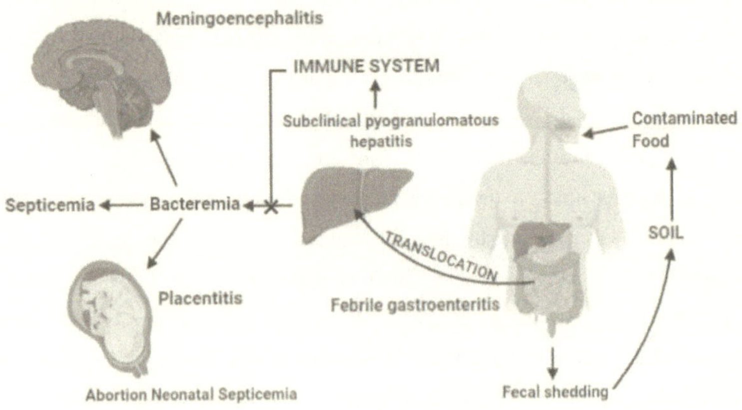

Figure 1. 3 Schematic pathophysiology of Listeria monocytogenes infection, showing some of the main organs affected and the effect on immunocompromised individuals, redrawn from (Vázquez-Boland *et al.* 2001)

1.2.1 *Listeria monocytogenes* History

Initially, *Lm* was discovered in the blood of laboratory rabbits and was named *Bacterium monocytogenes* by E.G.D Murray in 1924 since it could not be allocated to any pathogen genus at the time (Murray *et al.* 1926). It was only named *L. monocytogenes* in 1940 after confirmation as a Gram-positive rod by a catalase test (Pirie 1940). It was recognised as a significant foodborne pathogen, when a series of outbreaks started occurring in the USA and Europe in the 80s, thereafter, there have been other cases described worldwide (Schlech *et al.* 1983; Linnan *et al.* 1988; Miettinen *et al.* 1999). mortality rates of up to 30% have been recorded notwithstanding the availability of many antibiotics to treat *Lm* (Hamon *et al.* 2006). *Lm* can cross the blood-brain barrier, the placenta, also infecting organs such as the liver, spleen, the blood causing septicemia and minigitis. In South africa, there have been recent (2017 and 2018), large-scale outbreaks, which remains the largest to date (Desai *et al.* 2019). Several outbreaks in recent times with more than 950 confirmed cases, in certain circumstances mortality, reached 27%. These figures are comparable to outbreaks of other food borne diseases like *E coli* and *Salmonella*, though infectious is less lethal than *Lm*. (World Health Organization (WHO) 2018)

Lm uses the host machinery to enter various tissues and spread from cell to cell, invading non-phagocytic cells; like endothelial, epithelial, hepatic and phagocytic cells like macrophages and dendritic cells (Pamer 2004) (Figure 1.4). The internalin (Inl) genes InlA and InlB and p60 are used to gain entry into the various cells, once inside, the host surface receptors like E-cadherin, mesenchymal-epithelial transition factor (Met) and hepatocyte growth factor (HGF), component of extracellular matrix (ECM), and fibronecyin, entry is also facilitated by host opsonin-dependent pathway using the Fc gamma receptor (FcγR)/C3bi/C1q complement receptor (Edelson & Unanue 2001) In the opsonin-dependent pathway, *Lm* becomes coated with immunoglobulins IgG and C3bi/C1q complements in the bloodstream, which has the ability to interact with extracellular matrix proteins like collagens and fibronectin. This anchors on the cell wall of the host by IgG and C3bi/C1 and facilitates their uptake (Kwiatkowska & Sobota 1999). In the absence of serum, *Lm* is taken up, an indication of a nonopsonic macrophage scavenger receptor-ligand might be involved (Dunne *et al.* 1994; Greenberg *et al.* 1996; Vázquez-Boland *et al.* 2001). In other pathways (serum independent), surface proteins of *Lm* adhere to extracellular matrix protein containing ∞-D-galactose in dendritic cells, while in macrophages it binds to the scavenger receptor leading to entry, through phospholipid metabolism of the actin, remodelling of the cytoskeleton and acceleration of membrane traffic (Vieira *et al.* 2002). Following entry inside the cell, most of the *Lm* pathogen is killed within the first hour by phagosome-lysosome fusion, nonetheless, 14% of the bacteria escape into the cytoplasm using listeriolysin-O (LLO) (Cossart *et al.* 1989). Mutations in LLO renders *Lm* less virulent, limiting it into the cell for host killing. In other species like *Bacillus subtilis* LLO expression enables it to escape host vacuole (Stachowiak *et al.* 2012). Furthermore, purified LLO at certain pH dissolves the vacuole, demonstrating an important role of LLO in *Lm* virulence (Bielecki *et al.* 1990; Lee *et al.* 2009). Once escaped into the cytosol, the host actin protein is hijacked by the bacteria protein ActA for motility. (Figure 1.4) ActA is used to spread from cell to cell with the speed of movement determined by the concentration of protein actin, cell type, and environment. Lecithinase gene Phosphoryl-choline phospholipase A and B (*pcl*A and *pcl*B) are involved in the movements to adjacent cells after secondary invasion (Vazquez-Boland *et al.* 1992). The role of ActA gene was described when mutant Tn917-lac was defective for polymerization in tissue culture, bacteria could escape the vacuole but was unable move inside the cytoplasm. ActA gene alone is sufficient to mediate polymerisation-driven mobility of bacteria (Smith *et al.* 1995; Kocks *et al.* 1995) ActA uses the host cell machinery for *Lm* to move inside vacuole, it is responsible for the polymerization of actin tails. ActA performs this function mimicking the host actin nucleated factors like Wiskott–Aldrich syndrome protein (WASP) comprising Arp2/Arp3 complex, this complex is activated by VCA region of WASP. ActA also contain a VCA region which facilitates its capacity to polymerize the host actin for its movements .(Pizarro-Cerdá & Cossart 2006)

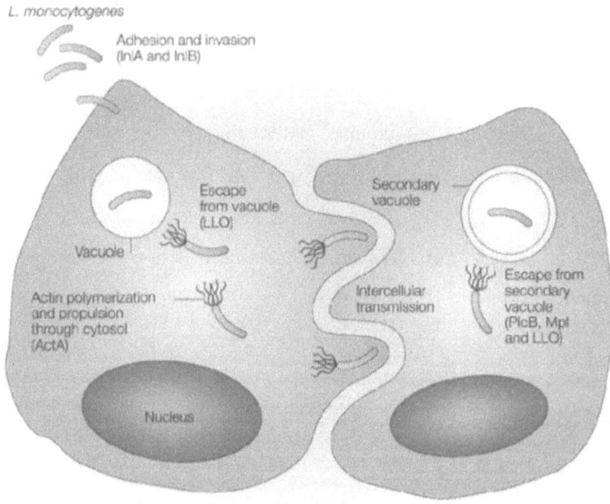

Figure 1. 4 Listeria monocytogenes, pathogenesis and cellular infection cellular and secreted proteins that enable attachment to the host. Listeriolysin-O (LLO) perforates phagosome membrane and escape into the cytosol, movement from cell to cell by the use ActA-dependent tail. Image from (Pamer 2004)

Lm uses InlA/B to subvert its host by avoiding non-phagocytic cells for easy persistence and evade immune activation. This enables it to multiply unabated, and secure a relatively safe niche (Cossart & Helenius 2014). During entry InlB which contains leucine-rich repeats, binds and stimulate the host proteins HGF and Met, leading to activation and proliferation and signalling through phosphatidylinositol 3-kinase (PI3K) and Ras-mitogen-activated protein kinase (MAPK) pathways eventually leading to entry into the host (Shen *et al.* 2000). Binding of InlB to E-cadherin recruits Arp2/3 complex which functions in creating new actin branches by nucleating new actin filaments. Arp2/3 complex activation is mediated by cortactin (Helwani *et al.* 2004). Cortactin recruits Rac1, a GTPase family member, *Lm* then triggers Rac1, which controls Arp2/3 complex facilitating cortactin translocation to *Lm* entry sites (Sousa *et al.* 2007). This process is as a result of InIA/B "mimicking' of homophilic E-adherin to initiate the activation of Rac1. InLB has also been shown to mimic the ligand hepatocyte growth factor(HGF), Met a tyrosine kinase receptor involved in mediating the proliferation and motility (Ferraris *et al.* 2010) InIA initiates Src-mediated tyrosine phosphorylation of E-cadherin, leading to ubiquitination by the cbl-like ubiquitin ligases (Bonazzi *et al.* 2008) which recruits clathrin-coated pits, thereby enabling the recruitment of actin. Therefore, InIA/InIB takes advantage of E-cadherin and the HGF-met mediated signalling pathways for its entry into the host (de Souza Santos & Orth 2015).

ListeriolysinO (LLO) functions better in an acidic milieu (pH 4.5-6.5), with optimal activity at pH5.5, an ideal pH to preserve LLO in the vacuole and enable escape into the cytosol (Glomski *et al.* 2002). Infected cells are protected from LLO in the phagosome and interact with the cell membrane and become neutralised with the high pH. This activity of LLO to change according to environment and pH, makes it better adapted to hijack and escape the phagosome from phagocytic killing.

ActA uses the host cell machinery for *Lm* to move inside vacuole, it is responsible for the polymerization of actin tails. ActA performs this function mimicking the host actin nucleated factors like Wiskott–Aldrich syndrome protein (WASP) comprising Arp2/ Arp3 complex, this complex is activated by VCA region of WASP. ActA also contains a VCA region which facilitates its capacity to polymerize the host actin for its movements (Pizarro-Cerdá & Cossart 2006) *Lm* has other mechanisms used to hijack and subvert host cellular machinery for entry, escape from the phagosome and movement to infect other cells not discussed here.

1.2.2 Host Killing and immune Responses to *Lm*

Like most other pathogens, the innate immune response plays a primordial role towards the elimination of *Lm* during initial infection, this role is usually non-specific, and it is the prelude for the adaptive immunity in case of insufficient clearance. The major phagocytic cells involved are neutrophils, resident macrophages, and natural killer (NK) cells. The role of innate immunity has been demonstrated in Severe Combined Immuno deficient (SCID) mice, lacking functional B and T cells, and nude mice, with no adaptive immunity. These mice are able to control *Lm* during the early stages but fail during the adaptive immunity phase (Bancroft *et al.* 1991), which is cell-mediated mainly by CD8 T cytotoxic cells lysing *Lm* (Bancroft *et al.* 1991; Unanue 1997). The liver and spleen are the first immune organs against *Lm* which are the first targets in preventing sepsis and dissemination and clear the pathogen by circulating resident macrophages. In the liver, the kupffer cells increase and are bactericidal, depletion of kupffer cells has been shown to increase bacilli burdens (Gregory & Wing 2002). Apart from these cells, there are some important cytokines and chemokines that are produced by innate cells IL-1, IFN-γ, IL-6, IL-10 TNF, IL-12, IL-18, MIP-2, (MIP)-1α, MIP-1β that are important for host killing of *Lm*.(Andersson *et al.* 1998; Brombacher *et al.* 1999; Lochner *et al.* 2008; McIlwain *et al.* 2012; Hoge *et al.* 2013). Resident macrophages do not kill all bacilli by phagolysosome fusion, the remaining bacteria in the liver grows in the hepatocytes (Cousens & Wing 2000; Zimmerer *et al.* 2016), *Lm* enters the parenchyma by two methods; uptake by kupffer cells, and by the hepatocytes using InIB and Met receptor (Shen *et al.* 2000) inhibiting the dead of host cell. Neutrophils are the first responder cells in most extracellular bacterial pathogens. During *Lm,* neutrophils are crucial for its control, early depletion of neutrophils using anti-GR1 and monoclonal antibody (RB6-8C5) have been shown to be detrimental in the control during infection. Though some studies show neutrophils playing no major role. The differences observed in different studies might be due to the route of administration of *Lm* and the target of the antibody (Shi *et al.* 2011). Besides neutrophils, inflammatory monocytes produce IL-12 and IL-15, and CCR2$^+$, two to four days after infection, monocytes replace neutrophils and in combinations to other cells congregate to form granuloma lesions, which preventing bacteria dissemination and eventual spread from cell to cell. NK cells produce IFN-γ necessary for macrophage and in combination with IL-6, TNF-α, IL-12 cytokines and inducible nitric oxide synthase (iNOS), ROS reactive oxygen (ROS) species which are key for clearance in macrophages to kill *Lm* by phagocytosis (Witter *et al.* 2016). Failure to adequately clear *Lm* by innate immune cells leads to *Lm*-specific T cells, activation is required to eliminate the bacterial and illicit T cell memory that offers protection during reinfection. T cells recruitment peaks from days 5 to 9 (Busch *et al.* 1998) CD4$^+$ T cells and CD8$^+$ T cells proliferate and differentiate independent of antigen, contribute towards cytokine production. (Mercado *et al.* 2000; Wong & Pamer 2001). CD8 T cells are the principal contributor in primary responses during *Lm* infection and most especially in secondary infection for protective immune memory responses (Pope *et al.* 2001). This has been confirmed by *in vivo* where depletion of CD8 T cells was shown to play a significant role (Czuprynski & Brown 1990; Kaufmann 1993). *Lm* peptides are presented either by major histocompatibility complex (MHC) MHC class I or MHC class II depending on the cell degradation of the peptide takes place either in the phagosome of the cytosol (Hiltbold & Ziegler 1993) When *Lm* gets inside the cytosol after escape from the vacuole, it is subjected to degradation by the proteasome. The peptides are loaded into MHC-I and presented to CD8$^+$ T cells (Wolf & Princiotta 2013). On the other hand, CD4$^+$ T cells are presented peptides degraded from the lysosomes and peptides presented by MHC-II. Cross presentation also takes place when antigens from the lysosome traffic into the endoplasmic reticulum and are loaded to MHC-I (Hiltbold & Ziegler 1993). CD8 T cells potentiate *Lm* immunity in two mechanisms which are synergistic, CD8 T cells secrete IFN-γ perforin and granzymes that lyse *Lm* infected cells thereby exposing them to macrophage targeted killing (Harty & Badovinac 2002). Pathogenicity of *Lm* is achieved by its ability to escape the phagosome into the cytosol using LLO (Berche *et al.* 1987). CD4 T cells play a lesser role than CD8 T cells during *Lm* infection. However, production of IFN-γ, TNF and IL-2, which are known to costimulate CD8 T cells in response to infection. (Shedlock *et al.* 2003). The role of CD4 T cells in *Lm* infection has been further confirmed by depletion experiments leading to susceptibility during infection (Romagnoli *et al.* 2017). During restimulation, memory T cells become activated and proliferate to control and eliminate *Lm*. This is achieved by the IFN-γ secretion by CD4 T cells that activate macrophages (Mouchacca *et al.* 2015). Perforin forms pores and is secreted by CD8 T cells and NK cells, it.is the most effective enzyme in clearing *Lm* during secondary infection (Harty *et al.* 1996). Mice deficient of perforin can control *Lm* during primary infection however, they succumb after re-challenged (Kägi *et al.* 1994). The function of perforin, granzyme B and other pro-inflammatory cytokines are influenced by many factors. Cytokines secreted by T reg are also known to affect cells around them and the type of cytokines there produce. Thus, understanding the relationship of T regulatory cells and *Lm* and the conditions that might influence their state and functions is important.

1.2.3 T Regulatory cells and *Lm*

Regulatory T cells secrete inhibitory cytokine including IL10 and TGF-β to dampen the activities of other T cells by immunosuppression. They are defined by the expression of $CD4^+CD25^+$ and the transcription factor Foxp3 (Hill *et al.* 2007). The role of T reg during *Lm* is not well studied. In one study, it was shown that during infection, immune expansion of T reg plays a detrimental role. This is so because T regs secrete inhibitory cytokines that depend on the effect of pro-inflammatory cytokines that are necessary for Th1 responses (Adalid-Peralta *et al.* 2011). Transient ablation of T regulatory cells has been shown to favour the rapid proliferation of $CD8^+$ T cells, which are necessary for protection against listeriosis (Harty & Badovinac 2002). Importantly, during pregnancy, T regs are known to expand up to 50% of their initial levels, this expansion is to maintain maternal tolerance to the foetus during pregnancy. (Ertelt *et al.* 2011) However, increase T regs have been shown to be detrimental during infection with *Lm* (Rowe *et al.* 2011). Transgenically induced T regs were shown to cause heightened susceptibility in infected mouse with *Lm* during pregnancy (Rowe *et al.* 2011). Maintenance of Foxp3 cells has been shown to be dose dependent during *Lm* infection. Low dose *Lm* induces a primary antigen-specific $CD8^+$ cytotoxic response dependent on $CD4^+$T cells. High dose *Lm* response is significantly inhibited by $CD4^+CD25^+FoxP3^+$ (Treg) (Dolina & Schoenberger 2017*b*). Similarly, the use of an LLO truncated human papillomavirus (HPV) based vaccine protein reduces the number of T reg cells (Gunn *et al.* 2001). Other studies show mutant attenuated *Lm* strain-based vaccine decreases the T reg with a corresponding increase in $CD4^+$ Foxp3$^-$ T cells, $CD8^+$ T cells by a mechanism dependent on LLO (Gunn *et al.* 2001). These studies suggest that T reg numbers and population affects the function of CD4 T cell and $CD8^+$ cytotoxic T cells during *Lm* infection. In mouse studies, transient ablation of Foxp3$^+$ T reg led to a corresponding increase in $CD8^+$ T cells leading to the protection during *Lm* (Rowe *et al.* 2011). However, this effect was not observed with recombinant *Lm* demonstrating that virulent *Lm* is required to elucidate protection and activate T regulatory cells proliferation (Ertelt *et al.* 2011). Splenic $CD8^+$ T cells expansion during infection leads to the secretion of key cytokines including IFN-γ, TNF and most importantly perforin potentiating in the effector killing function during infection. Even though these cytokines are also produced by other cells (NK cells and DCs, Mphs) (Harty & Badovinac

2002). CD8$^+$ T cells secrete more perforin than CD4$^+$ T cells that control of *Lm* growth. (Spaner *et al.* 1999).

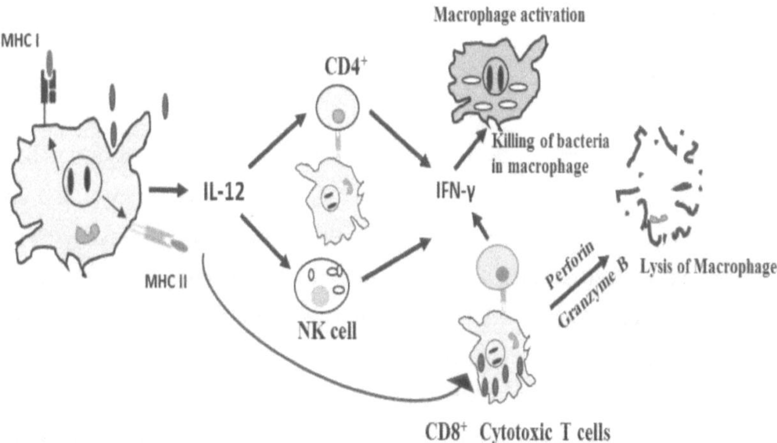

Figure 1. 5 Diagrammatic representation of macrophage activation and CD8+ T cell, the cytotoxic killing of *Listeria monocytogenes* with the production of IL-12 activation NK cells, CD4+ T cells and CD8+ T cells producing IFN-γ for direct killing or Cytotoxic killing by perforin and/or granzyme B.

Lm and *Mycobacterium tuberculosis* (*Mtb*) are both intracellular pathogens. *Mtb* remains one of the deadliest infectious pathogens, owing to its mechanism to hijack and evade host immune response. *Lm* has been widely used to understand host immune responses to identify genes against intracellular pathogens. *Lm* evades phagocytic and non-phagocytic cells to multiply and survive. Knowledge gained in *Lm* would be further studied in *Mtb*.

1.3 Tuberculosis

Tuberculosis (TB) is caused by *Mycobacterium tuberculosis* (*Mtb)* principally by airborne route between humans and is one of the greatest public health menaces with human immunodeficiency virus (HIV) as the major cause of death due to infectious diseases. There are medications for TB, the incidence, prevalence and mortality are still relatively stagnant.

Despite much efforts towards the elimination of the disease, TB still remains a major epidemic globally. TB mostly affects the poor and vulnerable populations disproportionately due to malnutrition, overcrowding and poor ventilation in houses. Current medications to TB are limited due to continuous development of drug-resistant forms thereby adding layers of complication in the available treatment options.

1.3.1 Brief History

TB has beset mankind for thousands of years. *Mycobacterium ulcerans* is thought to be of the Jurassic times causing human infections (Hayman 1984). Early progenitors of *Mtb* infected hominids were reported three million years ago in East Africa (Gutierrez *et al.* 2005). Early Egyptian arts and mummies dating 2400 BC with skeletal deformities and Pott's lesions that similar to *Mtb* infection (Morse *et al.* 1964; Zimmerman 1979). The old biblical testament has references to TB, during the time the Israelites lived in Egypt in the books of Deuteronomy and Leviticus (Daniel & Daniel 1999). Mortality rates of 900 per 100 000 inhabitants per year were recorded in 18th century Europe. In the 19th century, the description of phthisis attributing it to TB or a form of cancer as it was known then "cheese-like" abscesses (Houston 1999). In 1810, a French physician described disseminated form of TB known as "miliary" TB (Garrison 1921).

Early isolation of TB was cultured on egg white sterile flask, which turns muddy, this was recognised as mobile bacilli, which upon inoculation into Guinea pigs caused disease. Robert Koch used modern methods of methylene blue staining to identify the bacilli which remain a milestone in the fight against TB (Barberis *et al.* 2017). Charles Mantoux, Esmond R. Long and Florence Seibert developed the purified protein derivative (PPD) test base in Robert Koch tuberculin reaction (Barberis *et al.* 2017). In 1951, three research groups identified isoniazid as an anti-tuberculosis drug, the following year, Sir John Crofton introduced the use of tri-therapy with a combination of streptomycin, para-aminosalicyclic acid and isoniazid. Despite these advancements, TB remains a major health issue.

1.3.2 Epidemiology of TB

According to WHO, about 10 million people fell ill due to TB in 2018, with 1.6 million dead as a result of the disease, TB is also the primary killer among people with HIV. One Million Children develop TB with about 230 000 and died of the disease in the same year. A major blow to TB treatment is the emergence of multidrug-resistance (MDR-TB) with 558 000 new cases of resistance to rifampicin, which remains the most effective first-line drug treatment. Extensive drug resistance is also gaining grounds, defined as extreme drug resistance including one fluoroquinolone, and kanamycin, capreomycin and amikacin. Though the incidence of TB is dropping globally at 2% per year, the milestone target of 4-5% by 2020 is still farfetched. Most of the mortality due to TB occurs in developing countries, India, Russia, Ukraine, the Philippines, and China accounts for more than 40%. Tobacco consumption and HIV are a major risk factor to increase the risk of active TB (WHO 2018).

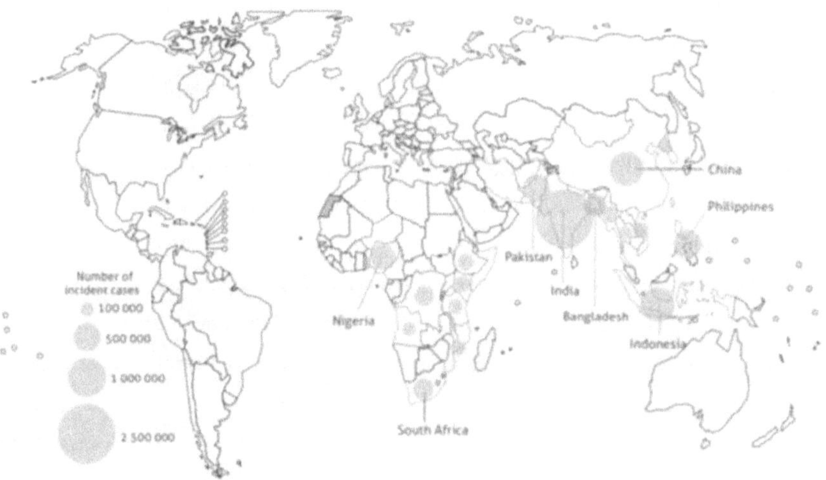

Figure 1. 6 Representation of TB high-burden countries: Nigeria, South Africa and DR Congo being the most affected in Africa (https://www.who.int/tb/publications/global_report/en/)

1.3.3 Immunopathology of TB

TB is transmitted mostly by droplets that contain the bacteria from people to people. The human immune system can, in most cases control the infection but does not lead to sterilization, these individuals are asymptomatic and are referred to as latently infected individuals (Horsburgh & Rubin 2011). These individuals are estimated to represent one-third of the global population, which might represent a potential reservoir. Also, 5-10% of these individuals subsequently develop TB in their lifetime. Resident lung alveolar macrophages are among the first cells for the immune defence, recruitment of other innate immune cells can lead to clearance, though this mechanism is not well (Cooper *et al.* 2011). Macrophages and their environmental factors determine the outcome of infection. The ability of macrophages to display plasticity and flexibility is important for the immune killing function. Macrophages transcription and function to a classical or alternative activation depending on the stimuli, during *Mtb* infection. Classical activation is activated with the release of pro-inflammatory cytokines like TNF, IL-12 and IL-1β, which requires control by alternative cytokine release necessary for wound healing (Mosser & Edwards 2008) In humans, alveolar macrophages do not meet this dichotomy during steady-state, they are 'hoovering' for cellular debris and ready for pro-inflammatory response during invasion (Hussell & Bell 2014). In non-human primate, a collection of cells immune cells during *Mtb* infection known as granuloma function differently. Balancing of classical and alternative activated macrophages is essential for the success of granuloma, with alternative activation playing a role in dampening inflammation but in the process also inhibit effective bacteria-killing (Flynn *et al.* 2011). Cytokines play a major role in the outcome of *Mtb* infection, there has an interplay with the induction of the adaptive arm and the "cross-talking" at the draining lymph nodes. Cytokines produced during the early stages of the disease also enables the initial formation of aggregates of innate cells, and later specialised cell types forming granuloma which are the hallmark of TB, these cells include T cells, B cells, neutrophils, NK cells, epithelioid macrophages, macrophages, foam cell, dendritic cell, and giant cells (Ndlovu & Marakalala 2016). The sequential accumulation of specialized cells determines the outcome of infection. Their nature and structure determine the release of cytokines and chemokines by activated macrophages in the granuloma (Flynn *et al.* 2011). Monocytes are also recruited from the bloodstream to the lungs and further differentiation into macrophages. Dendritic cells arrive as professional antigen presenters picking up *Mtb* antigens for or dead cells that have been phagocytised or dying cells by efferocytosis. This initial phase might lead to the control of *Mtb* by the innate immunity with negative tuberculin skin test (TST) or interferon-gamma release assay (IGRA) results, after repeated exposure to *Mtb*. The adaptive immune arm is activated by the priming from dendritic cells leading to T cell differentiation and proliferation. $CD4^+$ T cells play a key role by producing IFN-γ, IL-2, and TNF cytokines in response to *Mtb* infection. Other important cells are $CD8^+$ T cells, Th-17 cells, B cells and other non-canonical T cells (CD1 restrictive T cells, iNKT cells, γδ T cells, Mucosal associated invariant T cells) though not indispensable plays appreciated role in TB control (Kaufmann 2002; Nunes-Alves *et al.* 2014). The adaptive immunity leads to strong memory response by T cells with a positive TST and IGRA test. Some patients would be positive in TST and IGRA with no clinical symptoms referred to as subclinical TB but will be positive for culture, whereas active pulmonary patients will develop clinical symptoms including cough, fever, weight loss and will be TST, IGRA positive, culture-positive, sputum smear-positive or negative (Pai *et al.* 2016).

The T cell population and their plasticity can be exploited for host directed therapy. The IL-4Rα is a canonical receptor that defines Th2 disease response, through interaction with its ligand IL-4 and IL-13. The role of IL-4Rα and TB has not been widely studied.

1.3.4 Interleukin 4 Receptor alpha (IL-4Rα) and TB

The role of IL-4Rα and IL-4 in TB pathogenesis is contentious with opposing literature on the effect on granuloma and advancement to TB both in humans and mice studies. IL4 and IL-13 both signal through the IL-4Rα receptor, using the STAT-6 signalling, which is critical for the signalling and differentiation of naïve T cells into Th2 and secretion of IL-13/IL-4 (Wills-Karp & Finkelman 2008). Mouse model studies with global knockout of IL-4 on a C57BL/6 background, when infected with BCG, demonstrated that IL-4 was not decisive with no differences in bacterial burden and histopathology (Murray & Young 1999). Similarly, Mice deficient with the IL-4Rα in C57BL/6 mice also showed comparable bacterial load during *Mtb* infection (North 1998). This suggests that IL-4Rα in C57BL/6 background is not indispensable during *Mtb* infection. However, in BALB/c mice, one study showed no differences in bacteria burden when STAT-6 was deleted to skew the Th1/Th2 balance towards a Th1, despite the, increase in host protective IL-12, IFN-γ and iNOS, which likely contributed in histopathological differences. This study further showed that IL-4Rα$^{-/-}$ and IL-4/IL-13$^{-/-}$ mice had similar growth of *Mtb* in the lungs, liver and spleen (Jung *et al.* 2002). Previously, our laboratory demonstrated that specific deletion of IL-4Rα on macrophages/neutrophils (LysM^{cre}IL-4Rα$^{-/lox}$) in mice resulted in comparable mortality, bacterial burden, histopathology and no differences in iNOS and Arginase (Arg1) following infection with hyper virulent HN878 strain of *Mtb* (Guler *et al.* 2015).

Other studies using a neutralising anti-IL-4 polyclonal or monoclonal antibody in BALB/C mice showed differences with decreased CFUs in tissues when anti IL-4 and anti-IL-13 was used (Buccheri *et al.* 2007) A possible explanation in these differences might be a compensation mechanism or lack of proper development in IL-4/IL-4Rα mice. Mice with transient deletion, therefore, was better suitable in this case (Roy *et al.* 2008). In BALB/C mice, IL-4 had a modestly harmful effect on the Th1 immune response with increased TNF and fibrosis (Hernandez-Pando *et al.* 2004). In asthma models of mice and, IL-4 inhibition using monoclonal antibody led to rapid clearance of *Mtb* (Hart *et al.* 2002). Pre-existing *Nippostrongylus brasiliensis* (*Nb*) (predispose animals to Th2 immune responses) infection, shows impaired resistance to *Mtb* infection in mouse, suggesting a link where TB and helminthic infections coexist. Co-infected mice with deletion IL-4Rα$^{-/-}$ and *Nb* infection displayed better ability to control *Mtb* infection (Potian *et al.* 2011). In humans, increase lung cavity granuloma has been shown to be related to increased expression of IL-4 during the progression of the disease (van Crevel *et al.* 2000). Also, mRNA transcriptional expression of IL-4 increases during active pulmonary TB in the lungs (Dheda *et al.* 2007). Another study showed an increase in IL-4Rα mRNA expression in PBMCs (Schauf *et al.* 1993). A house contact study of individuals in contact with active TB patients validated the association of IL-4/IL-4Rα and TB patient with increase expression of IL-4Rα in both groups upon contact (Mihret *et al.* 2013). IL-4 and IL-13 are structurally and functional similar cytokines, much has been studied on IL-4/IL-4Rα but not IL-13 and TB. IL-13 over-expression in BALB/c background after infection with H37RV strain resulted in significant increase in(Heitmann *et al.* 2014) pulmonary granulomas. suggest that IL-4/IL-4Rα might be associated with active pulmonary TB. These association and their outcome are not fully understood in the different cellular population.

1.3.5 Foxp3 T regulatory cells and TB

Mtb establishes persistent infections that may require mechanisms that check excessive immunological responses. T reg plays a vital role in preventing autoimmunity, but also suppress antimicrobial immune responses. Understanding the role of Foxp3 T regs in TB only started in 2006 (Guyot-Revol *et al.* 2006; Quinn *et al.* 2006). The role of T reg has been studied in other models including *Leishmania major* where they play a role in inhibiting immune response during mouse infection. Depletion was shown to enhance clearance with increased effector T cell function CD4$^+$CD25$^-$ (Belkaid *et al.* 2002). *Mtb* is slow in activating the adaptive immunity compared to other pathogens, with infected individuals becoming positive from 6 weeks onwards (Wallgren 1948; Behr *et al.* 2018). In mouse models, this delay has been observed especially with the recruitment of T cells. (Urdahl *et al.* 2011). In normal circumstances, the early arrival of T cells is associated with clearance of *Mtb* in the lungs. This delay occurs at different phases, which includes, *Mtb*-infected DCs arrival in the draining lymph nodes, delay in effector expansion and migration to the lungs (Chackerian *et al.* 2002; Wolf *et al.* 2007, 2008; Reiley *et al.* 2008). In humans during the first weeks of infection, T reg is recruited to the lungs corroborated with a decrease in peripheral blood T reg cells (Burl *et al.* 2007). This was further confirmed in macaques as T reg was observed to migrate to the lungs during early infection (Green *et al.* 2010). Since we observe a delay in the arrival of CD4$^+$ T cells, and the early arrival of T regs, the role of T reg is detrimental during *Mtb* infection. We hypothesis that manipulation of T reg may affect the functionality and quality of T regs, thereby influencing the CD4$^+$ T cell effector balance. To achieve this, our laboratory generated mice lacking IL-4Rα specifically on Foxp3 T reg.

1.4 Generation of Foxp3$^+$ T regulatory cell-Specific IL-4Rα Knockout mice

The use of cell-specific knockout mice has been a very valuable tool in delineating the function of IL-4Rα signalling on various immune cells in different disease models. This has been achieved largely due to the novel methods of using the Cyclization (Cre) recombinase and LoxP (locus of X over P). IL-4Rα gene is flanked and either inverted or translocated using the enzyme Cre recombinase. The Cre is under the control of a specific cell type, in this case, Foxp3 promoter. These mice are crossed with IL-4Rα is flanked by lox-P transgenic mice. The offspring of these mice will have a deletion of the specific gene under this promoter by the Cre slicing at the lox-P sites. Using this technology, we have in the past generated a transgenic mouse that the exons 7 and 9 of the IL-4Rα flanked by the lox-P sites. IL-4Rα deletion of CD4 T cells (Leeto *et al.* 2006; Radwanska *et al.* 2007; Dewals *et al.* 2009) on B Cells (Hoving *et al.* 2012) on macrophages and neutrophils (Cao *et al.* 2007) Dendritic cells and alveolar macrophages (Hurdayal *et al.* 2013) and smooth muscle cells (Marillier *et al.* 2010). In order to understand the role of IL-4Rα signalling on key regulatory immune cells, T regs we generated IL-4Rα deletion on Foxp3 cells, with an intact receptor on all other immune cell populations.

1.5 Rationale

T-regulatory cells (Treg) have as main function the maintenance of self-tolerance and prevention of autoimmunity. However, they also play a crucial role in the homeostatic immune response due to pathogenic infection through regulation of inflammation (Smigiel *et al.* 2014). T reg is developed either from the thymus or from the periphery. Thymic T reg migrates to secondary lymphoid organs and tissues where they affect cytokines, expand and control tissue damage. The ability of T cells to differentiate to different types of lineages and their cytokine produced has been highly exploited for their therapeutic potential during infection or immunization through their manipulations (Parida *et al.* 2015) T reg cells (CD25$^+$CD4$^+$) have been shown to have diverse functions during ablation with different disease models. During *L. major* infection, for example, T reg accumulates within chronic sites of the skin with detrimental effects where they suppress effector cells by both IL-10-dependent and independent mechanisms (Belkaid *et al.* 2002). In parasitic infection of *Plasmodium berghei*, Foxp3$^+$ proliferation leads to protection in severe forms of malaria disease, demonstrating a beneficiary role (Haque *et al.* 2010).

During viral infection like in herpes simplex depletion of cell specific T reg cells led to enhanced CD8$^+$ T cell function; with proliferation and cytotoxicity (Suvas *et al.* 2003). Studies, where T regs have been depleted with the rebust transcriptional factor signature foxp3 rather than $CD4^+CD25^+$, have shown conflicting outcome in viruses, parasites, fungi, and bacteria. In herpes simplex virus 2, West Nile virus, lymphocytic choriomeningitis virus, $Foxp3^+$ cell ablation lead to increased viral load and subsequent mortality (Lund *et al.* 2008; Lanteri *et al.* 2009).

Similarly, during fungal infection with *Candida albicans*, adoptive transfer *of* $Foxp3^+$ Tregs into Rag deficient mouse (mice with no T and B cells) led protection compared to mouse receiving conventional T cells ($CD4^+CD25^-CD44^-$) (Pandiyan *et al.* 2011).

Paradoxically, in most bacterial infections notable *Salmonella enterica*, expansion of $Foxp3^+$ Tregs was found to be detrimental during pregnancy and increased bacterial burden (Johanns *et al.* 2010; Rowe *et al.* 2011). This outcome was similar in *Mycobacterium tuberculosis* infection in which decrease of $Foxp3^+$ cells in mixed chimera mice led to a decreased bacterial burden, transfer of $Foxp3^+$ cells reduced the effector's arm and hence decreased killing and subsequent more bacterial burden (Scott-Browne *et al.* 2007; Shafiani *et al.* 2010). Similarly, in *Lm* infection, Foxp3 cell proliferation resulted in exacerbated bacterial burden due to dampening of the effector T cells, is was overturned by $Foxp3^+$ cell deletion (Rowe *et al.* 2011).

Considering the important role T regs play in maintaining immune tolerance, specific manipulation of this population in response to molecular cues such as cytokines and cofactors has been a promising approach for treatment for communicable and non-communicable diseases (Sawant *et al.* 2012; Jin *et al.* 2013; Ulges *et al.* 2015). This can be achieved by cytokines, that have reportedly played a critical role in the functions of T reg. Interferon-γ (IFN-γ) secretion, Foxp3 T reg cells upregulates the Th1 specific transcriptional factor T-bet (Koch *et al.* 2009) Other cytokines like IL-2 shut down T regs contributing to a Th1 environment, TGF-beta and IL-6 driving the expression of $Foxp3^+$ T reg (Bettelli *et al.* 2007; Campbell & Koch 2011). Th2 cytokines have also been shown to play a role in the development and function of T reg cells IL-4 through the STAT-6/GATA-3 expression leading to decreased levels of T reg converting to a Th2 during type 2 diseases (Wang *et al.* 2010; Hansmann *et al.* 2012). IL-4 signals through IL-4 receptor alpha (IL-4Rα) during type 2 diseases, deleting this specific receptor signalling on $Foxp3^+$ T reg cells, might shift the Tregs/Th2 balance to an effector Th1. Methodical increase of IL-4Rα signalling on T regs showed reprogrammation into Th2 lineage (susceptible) while deletion led to protection during food allergy (Noval Rivas *et al.* 2015). In a recent study, a mutation on IL-4Rα on Tregs cells led to a Th-17 lineage (Massoud *et al.* 2016). The role of IL-4Rα on CD4$^+$Foxp3$^+$ regulatory T cells was further demonstrated during *H polygyrus* a Th2 model. IL-4 signalling through IL-4Rα was required to control *H polygyrus*, by the convertion of T regs to Th2 cells (Pelly *et al.* 2017). Therefore, during infection, since Th2 are essential for the control of *H. polygyrus* IL-4Rα presence on T reg is an important component for plasticity to occur. Recently our laboratory, reported the role of specific deletion of IL-4Rα on Foxp3 regulatory cells in *S. mansoni* infection Obliteration led to exercebated tissue damage and excessive inflammation at the liver, due to disfunction of the Foxp3$^+$ Treg cells accompanied by uncontrolled effector T cells (Aziz *et al.* 2018). In addition, we have found that IL-4Rα signalling on Foxp3 T reg is necessary for the control of allergic responses during House dust mite allergen (in revision). These studies highlighted the role of IL-4Rα in Th2 models. The effect of the IL-4Rα in Th1 models has not been well elucidated. In this study, our aim was to determine the effect of IL-4Rαdeletion on Foxp3$^+$ T reg cell in T helper 1 (Th1) infecction models. Therefore, the aim of this study was to understand the impact of this receptor signalling in driving the outcome of listeriosis and tuberculosis.

1.5.1 Hypothesis

We hypothesized that specific deletion of IL-4Rα on FoxP3$^+$ T Regulatory cells affects the quality FoxP3$^+$ T Regulatory cells hence rendering them prone to enhanced Th1 effector response in mouse model of listeriosis and tuberculosis

1.5.2 Objectives of this study

(A) To determine the effect of specific deletion of IL-4Rα on FoxP3$^+$ Tregs on the immune regulation during *Listeria monocytogenes* infection in mice

(B) To determine the effect of IL-4Rα signalling on FoxP3$^+$ Tregs during *Mycobacterium tuberculosis* infection in mice

CHAPTER 2:
MATERIALS AND METHODS

Methods

2.1 Mouse strain

Deletion of *il-4rα* gene in Foxp3-expressing cells (Foxp3[cre] IL-4Rα$^{-/lox}$) BALB/c mice were generated as previsouly described (Aziz *et al.* 2018). Briefly, Foxp3[cre]IL-4Rα$^{-/lox}$ was produced by crossing a Cre BALB/c mice with *foxp3* gene promoter and IL-4Rα$^{-/-}$ BALB/C mice for two generations and then further crossed with floxed IL-4Rα (IL-4Rα$^{-/lox}$) BALB/c mice to specifically delete IL-4Rα exons 7 and 9 on flanked sites of Foxp3$^+$ T reg. Mice were housed in the specific-pathogen free (SPF) animal facility of Faculty of Health Sciences, University of Cape Town.

2.2 Ethics Statement

All experiments with animals and protocols were performed in strict accordance with the South African National Standards, as well as the Animal Research Ethics Committee (AEC No. 015/037 for Listeria and 015/040 for *Mtb*) of the Faculty of Health Sciences, University of Cape Town project. Considerations for the humane ending of the sick mouse was highly respected and adhered during the course of the study by all involved in the project.

2.3 *Listeria monocytogenes* culture and infection

Stock solutions of *Lm* (virulent EGD strain) were maintained by mouse passaged in BALB/c mouse and grown in a medium of Tryptic-Soy Broth (TSA)(Difco) at 37° C and harvested at a mid-log phase of (O.D$_{600}$=0.3-0.6). Harvested *Lm* was stored in glycerol (%) stocks, at -80°C for further use. To determine the stock concentration, serial dilutions were plated on Tryptic soy agar (TSA) plates for 24 hours (Dai *et al.* 1997). During each experiment, the concentration was determined by platting before and after infection on a TSA plate at 10-fold dilutions. For mortality infections, $2x10^5$ *Lm*/200µl was used and $2x10^4$ *Lm*/200µl for time course experiments at 3 and 7 days post infections (dpi). Foxp3[cre]IL-4Rα$^{-/lox}$ and littermate controls where vaccinated with low *Lm* ($1x10^4$) and re-challenged with 100 fold dose 30 days after. All *Lm* infections were done intra-peritoneally in 200µl volume of PBS using 1ml insulin syringe.

2.4 *Mycobacterium tuberculosis* culture and infection

Mtb strain H37Rv was BALB/c passaged to maintain virulence and aerosol inhalation mimicking the natural route of *Mtb* infection. Few colonies where picked and grown on a 7H10 Middlebrook broth (Difco-Detroit-MI, USA) with the addition of Middlebrook OADC enrichment medium (Sigma-Aldrich Darmstadt, Germany). A total of $2x10^6$ live bacteria was suspended in 6ml PBS solution to obtain a low dose of 100 CFU/lung upon arerosol passage using the glass-col nebulising aerosol inhalation system at the BSL3 Animal Facility Unit. The dose was confirmed a day later by plating 250µl on 7H10 Middlebrook plates prepared with PANTA (polymixin B, amphotericin, nystatin, trimethoprim, azlocillin). (PANTA; Becton, Dickinson and Company, Spark, USA)

2.5 Mouse monitoring after infection

After infection, mice were monitored twice daily for *Lm* infection and once daily for *Mtb*-infected mice. Mice that had lost more than 20% of their initial body weight or presented with a severe illness accompanied and/or behavioural changes like hunched back posturing, lack of grooming where declared moribund and euthanized.

2.6 Bacterial burden determination

For both *Lm* and *Mtb* infections, bacterial load were determined at various time points. Organs were collected in an aseptic manner and divided into three portions (Bacterial burden, histology and FACS). Every organ was weight accordingly to determine the propotional bacterial burden per organ. Tissue portions were homogenised in 1X PBS with 0.05% Tween-80. Homogenates were serially diluted in a 10-fold in 1X-PBS and 100µl plated in TSA plates for *Lm* and on 7H10 agar plates for *Mtb*. Plates were incubated for 37°C for 24hours (*Lm*) and 17-21 days for *Mtb* colony counting.

2.7 Tissue Histopathology

For each experiment, consistent portions of spleen or lobes of the liver were collected for *Lm* and lungs for *Mtb* infection. Fixed with 4% formalin and rehydrated with Xylol and alcohol during the preparation of slides. Three different cuts (2-3µm) were obtained in each mouse for hemotoxylin and eosin (H&E) staining for pathological and immune cell infiltration and lesion sizes. The acquisition was done using the Nikon Eclipse 90i Microscope. Analysis and visualization of alveolar air spaces were determined using the software Nikon NIS element.

2.8 Enzyme-linked immunosorbent Assay (ELISA)

Concentrations of the various cytokine and chemokines (IL-12p40, IL-12p70, IL-23, IL-6, TNF, IL-1α, IL-1β, IFN-γ, IFN-β, IL-17, Igf-1, IL-10, IL-4, TGF-β, GM-CSF, M-CSF, CCL2, CCL3, CXCL1, CXCL10, CXCL2 and CXCL5) were carried out by ELISA. Liver homogenates, spleen re-stimulation, and serum for *Lm*; lung homogenates samples for *Mtb* infection. Sandwiched ELISA was performed on Nunc Maxisorp flat-bottom 96 well plates (Roskilde, Denmark) coated with the various antibodies and blocking with 2% BSA. Biotinylated detection of secondary antibodies where used according to their cytokines to be detected. Horseradish peroxidase (HRP) or alkaline phosphatase (AP) with PNP (4-nitrophenyl disodium salt-hexahydrate) (dilution: 0.05g in 50ml) substrate solution (Sigma Aldrich) was used. H_2SO_4 at 1M was used to stop the reaction. An absorbance of 405 nm was used on the SoftMax program.

2.9 Nitric Oxide Measurement

Lung supernatants were used to measure the concentration of Nitric Oxide (NO) by Griess reaction assay. Standards (Na_2NO_3, 2mM) were prepared at a starting concentration of 0.1M with a two-fold serial dilution in triplicates on NUNC flat bottom 96 well plate. 50µL of samples were added followed by adding of 25µL reagent A (1% sulfanilamide($C_6H_8N_2O_2S$) in 2.5% phosphoric acid (H_3PO_4) incubated for 5 mins at room temperature and then 25µL reagent B (0.1% napthyl ethylenediamine in 2.5% phosphoric acid). Further, incubated in the dark for 5-10 mins. When a purple colour was visible relative to the standards the reaction was stopped with 100µL of 96% H_2SO_4/85% H_3PO_4 /85% H_2O. Plates were read at 540 nm with reference of 690 nm.

2.10 Isolation and stimulation of mediastinal lymph node

The mediastinal lymph node was harvested from mice and passed through a 70µM followed by 40µM strainer to obtain single-cell suspensions. Cells were centrifuged at 1200 rpm for 10 mins at 4° C. Single cells were resuspended in 2ml complete Dulbecco's Modified Eagle's Medium (DMEM, Gibco) supplemented with 10% FCS, viable cells were counted with Trypan Blue (0.4%). A total of 2×10^6 cells were seeded in 100µl media and left unstimulated, or stimulated with H37Rv Lysate at 10µg/ml, or 50ng/ml PMA, 250 ng/ml ionomycin combined with 200 µM monensin, for 8 hours. Immuno-staining was done with 50µl antibody mix with 2% rat serum and 10µg FcγRI

2.11 Real-Time PCR

Total RNA was extracted with mini-elute columns according to the manufacturer's protocol. (Qiagen, http://www.quiagen.com) from splenocyte and hepatocytes after infection at different time points. RNA quality was determined using NanoDrop 200. cDNA was obtained by transcription using first stranded cDNA Synthesis Kit (Roche). The random hexamer primer and anchored oligo dT primers were used with respect to the manufacturer's instructions Quantitative Real-time PCR was done with LightCycler® 480 SYBR Green I Master mix in LightCycler® 480 II (Roche). *HPRT* was used as the normalization gene for absolute quantifications (Silver *et al.* 2008).

2.12 Data extracted from public available transcriptomic studies

Public available cohort studies (Mahomed *et al.* 2011; Thompson *et al.* 2017) RNA data was obtained from the blood of quantiferon negative (healthy), latently and tuberculosis patients. Transcriptional signatures from prospective cohorts data of active TB cases controlled BCG[+] cases were plotted from South Africa, (Malawi and united Kingdom) (Maerten *et al.* 2005; Berry *et al.* 2010; Mahomed *et al.* 2011; Bloom *et al.* 2013; Cliff *et al.* 2013; Kaforou *et al.* 2013; Dawany *et al.* 2014; Zhai *et al.* 2015; Thompson *et al.* 2017). Latent TB was defined by the tuberculin skin test or QuantiFERON Gold test. Active TB was defined as two or more sputum-smears positive for the acid fast test or one positive cultured sputum for M. tuberculosis.

2.13 Primers used for murine cell population

Primers for quantitative RT-PCR of IL-4Rα and Foxp3	
Gene Target	Primer
FoxP3- Forward	5'-CTGCCACCTGGGATCAATGT-3'
FoxP3- Reverse	5'- GGCAGAGCCCTTCCGCACTT-3'
IL-4Rα-Forward	5'-ACTGGATCTGGGAGCATAAA-3'
IL-4Rα-Reverse	5'-CCTATTCATTTCCATGTGGCA-3'
HPRT – Forward	5'-GGCCATGAGGCTGGATCTC-3'
HPRT -Reverse	5'-AACATTTGAATCCTGCAGCCA-3'

2.14 Flow Cytometry

Extracellular staining was perfomed on cell population by seeding 2×10^6 cells per well in a 96 well NUNC plate in FACS buffer. Centrifuged at 1200 rpm for 5 mins at 4° C. Stained with 50µL of antibody cocktail [Myeloid panel, CD11C-FITC (clone:HL3), Gr-1-APCcy7(Clone:RB6-8C5) MHCII-APC(Clone:M5/114.15.2), F4/80Pecy7 (Clone:BM8)] [Lyphmphocyte panel CD3-A700 (clone500A2) CD8-V500(S3-6.7)) CD44-FITC (cloneIM7), CD62L-V4509 (clone MEL-14), CD19-APCCy7(cloneID3),CD4-Percp (cloneRM4-5),CD124-PE (cloneG077F6)]. 1% of heat-inactivated rat serum and 10 µg/ml anti-FcR blocking FcγII and FcγIII receptors was added. Incubated for 30-35 minutes at 4°C, and resuspended in FACS buffer. Further spun down and fixed with 2% paraformaldehyde in PBS, and resuspended in 200µL of FACS buffer for acquisition. Surface makers of myeloid cells and T cells were acquired using the BD LSRFortessa™.

Intra-cellular(IC) cytokine staining was carried out by first surface staining, then washed with FACS buffer, centrifuged at 1200 rpm for 5 mins and permeabilised with permeabilisation buffer (Invitrogen Life Technologies), for 45-60 minutes in the dark at 4°C. Staining was done in 50 µl cytokine Ab cocktail (Ab against different cytokines + (1x 2%iRBS+ 1% 4.2G2)). Intracellular cytokines were stained with IL-2-FITC (cloneJES6-5H4), IFNγ-A700 (cloneXMG1.2), IL-17-PercyCy5.5 (cloneEbIO17b7), IL-4-PE(clone 11B11), IL-10 (clone JES052A5).

Intra-nuclear(IN) staining was performed similarly to IC, briefly after extracellular staining, cells were conditioned with Fixation- Permeabilization wash buffer. Permeabilised by incubating for 1hr at 4°C using permeabilization buffer for, FoxP3-APC (cloneMF23), Ki67-PE (cloneB56), BCL-2FITC (clone3F11), Caspace3-PE (Clone C92-605), GranzymeB V450 (cloneGB11) , GATA3-Percy (Clone TWAJ).

The acquisition was achieved using the LSRFortessa™ (BD Immunocytometry Systems, San Jose, CA, USA). All generated data from the Fortessa were analysed using Flowjo software (FlowJo v10.0.7) (Treestar, Ashland, OR, USA). See gating strategy at the supplementary figures.

2.15 In vitro macrophage coculture with CD4$^+$CD25$^-$ and CD4$^+$CD25$^+$

2.15.1 Bone marrow-derrived macrophage generation (BMDM)

Bone marrow-derrived macrophage (BMDM) were generated as described previously (Hölscher *et al.* 2006). Briefly, femurs were obtained from 8-12 weeks old male IL-4Rα$^{-/lox}$ BALB/c mice cultured for 10 days with L929-cell conditioned medium. L929-cells was a source of granulocyte and macrophage colony stimulating factor with DMEM supplemented with 10% fetal calf serum, 5% inactivated horse serum, 1% β-mercaptoethanol, 1mM sodium pyruvate, 1% 100U/ml penecillin, 100µg/ml streptomycin (Penstrep), and 2mM L-glutamine. (Gibco cat 12657-029). After 10 days, cells differentiation were confirmed by microscopy by their elongated morphological structure. Debris and non-adherence cells where washed with 1X PBS. The adherent cells were incubated with 1X PBS containing 5 mM EDTA and 4 mg/ml lidocaine for 10 mins. Cells were stained with Trypan blue to distinguish between dead and live cells and counted under a microscope using the NebHaur chamber. 25x10^5 cell/well was seeded on a round bottom plate for T cell co-culture.

2.15.2 *Lm* infection of BMDM

Seeded BMDMs cells were left overnight and infected with heat killed *Lm* (HKLM) at a multiplicity of infection (MOI) of 1:5 and incubated for 24 hours on CO_2 incubator for 24 hours at 37^0C.

2.15.3 Flow cytometry and FACS T cell sorting

Spleens were harvested from FoxP3^creIL-4Rα ^-/lox mice and littermate control mice. Single cell suspension to obtain splenocytes was achieved by disrupting spleens through a 40µm filter. Washed with DMEM+10% FCS. The cells were counted on the NebHauer Chamber using a brightfield microscope (Nikon Ecclipse). T cells sorting was performed using using BD FACSAria™ Fusion flow cytometer. FACS analysis was performed using BD LSRFortessa™ flow cytometer. Viable cells were determined using LIVE/DEAD BV605 (Thermofisher Scientific). Cells stained for CD3-A700, CD4-BV510, CD19-PerCp, and CD25-PE where used to obtain CD4$^+$CD25$^-$ and CD4$^+$CD25$^+$ cell population. Stained cells were fixed in 2% formaldehyde fro 30 minutes at 4°C.

2.15.4 BMDM co-culture of with T cells

CD4$^+$CD25$^-$ (effector) and CD4$^+$CD25$^+$ (T reg) T-cells were added to BMDMs (MØ) in a 48 well plate at different ratios [1 (MØ):1 (effector) / 1(MØ): 3 (effector) / 1(MØ): 3 (effector) : 1(T reg)]. Cells were incubated for 72 hours (3 days). After incubation, the supernatant was collected for cytokine ELISAs. Cells were lifted with 1X PBS in EDTA and lidocaine, washed and stained. Cells were stained extracllularly with CD4-BV510, CD62L-V450, CD44-FITC, KLRG1-BV786, F4/80-PEcy7, and intracellularly stained with Ki-67-PE, Foxp3-APC.

2.17 Statistics

All Data was analysed using Prism software (Prism software; Using either Student's *t*-test (two-tailed with unequal variance) or 1-way-ANOVA Dunnett's -post-test. Results are represented as mean ± SD. With statistical significant represented as (*, p 0.05; **, *p* 0.01; ***, p 0.001).

CHAPTER 3:
RESULTS

The aim of this study is to investigate the role of IL-4Rα on Foxp3 T regulatory cells during *Listeria monocytogenes* and *Mycobacterium tuberculosis* infections in mice. In this chapter, the results are presented in two sections. The first section describes infection with *Lm,* evaluating the differences in the protein levels of both Foxp3 and IL-4Rα, bacterial burden, mortality, cytokine dynamics at various tissues, histopathology and immune cell populations that are affected due to the loss of IL-4Rα on Foxp3$^+$ T regulatory cells. In the second section of the results, we infected mice with *Mtb* H37Rv strain infection to further understand the role IL-4Rα signalling plays during slow-growing bacteria infection in mouse models.

3.1 Section one

3.1.1 Abstract *Lm* infection

IL-4Rα signalling on Foxp3$^+$ regulatory T cells regulates immune response to *Listeria monocytogenes* infection

Cytokine signalling is a significant component influencing the control and function of Forkhead box P3 (Foxp3) CD4$^+$CD25$^+$ T regulatory cells (T reg), which are critical in the maintenance of self-tolerance, immune homeostasis and regulation of the immune system. IL-4Rα is the predominant canonical receptor through which IL-4 and IL-13 signals. Th2 dependent models utilize IL-4Rα signalling on the different cell populations. IL-4 responsive T regulatory cells signal through IL-4 Receptor alpha (IL-4Rα) has been widely studied in Th2 disease models. T regulatory cells are an integral immune cell population that suppresses overtly secreted cytokines during inflammation; however, this role can be detrimental during bacterial infections by suppressing Th1 responses needed for clearance. Specific manipulation of T regs by the deletion of IL-4Rα is a novel approach for Th1 disease settings. There is limited knowledge of IL-4Rα signalling on T regulatory cells and impact on Th1 disease models. We generated Foxp3-specific IL-4Rα deficient (FoxP3^{cre}IL-4Rα$^{-/lox}$) mice through an X-linked Foxp3 promoter directed Cre recombinase activity. Using this mouse in an experimental model of listeriosis, we demonstrated that impairment of IL-4Rα–mediated signalling specifically within the Foxp3 T reg population resulted in significant difference in survival and decreased bacterial burden compared to the littermate control. This was further accompanied by smaller lesions sizes in the spleen and liver revealed by histopathological analysis. Flow cytometry analysis demonstrated enhanced effector T cells producing IFN-γ, IL-

2 and increased expression of T-bet transcription factor signature at 7 dpi. In addition, abrogated signalling of IL-4Rα on T regs showed an increase in CD8$^+$ T cells that produced granzyme B and IFN- γ necessary for killing of *Lm*. Furthermore, CD8$^+$ T cells showed increased proliferation by Ki67 staining, better survival by BCl-2 levels and decreased apoptosis by activated caspase-3 staining. Cytokines measured in the spleen upon restimulation with anti-CD3 and HKLM and sera revealed a pro-inflammatory environment with a significant increase in IFN-γ at 7dpi. Liver homogenate showed an increase in TNF, IL-10 and IL-4. Moreover, the co-culture of bone marrow-derived macrophages, T cells and T regs from Foxp3^{cre}IL-4Rα$^{-/lox}$ mice confirm an important role the receptor in T regs in the control of *Lm*. Together, these results show a novel role of IL-4 responsive T regulatory cells in host immunity *Lm* infection in mice.

3.1.2 IL-4Rα and Foxp3 mRNA expression during the progression of *Lm* infection in mice.

We compared the expression of IL-4Rα and Foxp3 mRNA during the course of 2 to 10 days of listeria infection in both spleen and liver. This enables us to determine first whether *Lm* infection regulates the IL-4Rα and Foxp3 expression as a function of time. BALB/c mice were infected with 2×10^4 *Lm* sub-lethal dose intraperitoneally; this route was chosen because the oral route has been shown to have lower reproducibility, and also requires a higher inoculum dose as validated by us and others (Gaillard *et al.* 1991). After infection, at 2, 5, 7 and 10 days, Il4rα mRNA transcript was consistently decreased in the spleen (Figure 3.1A), suggesting *Lm* infection down-regulate Il4rα expression. Similarly, Foxp3 transcript decreases significantly early after infection at day 2 and day 5, however, it starts increasing at day 7 and restored to the levels uninfected spleen by day 10(Figure 3.1B). Conincidently, at day 10 mice do clear the *Lm* infection around day10 (Wang *et al.* 2011).

In liver tissue, there was a transient increase in the expression of Il4rα up from naïve to 5 dpi and a decreased to the uninfected liver levels by day 10 (Figure 3.1C). In contrast to spleen, FoxP3 mRNA transcripts had no differences in the liver (Figure 3.1D). Therefore, Listeria infection modulates the of Il4rα expression, which reverts to naïve state at later stages of the infection. Furthermore, foxp3 expression signifiantly altered in spleen but not liver. These alterations in gene expression levels suggest that they are affected during *Lm* infection.

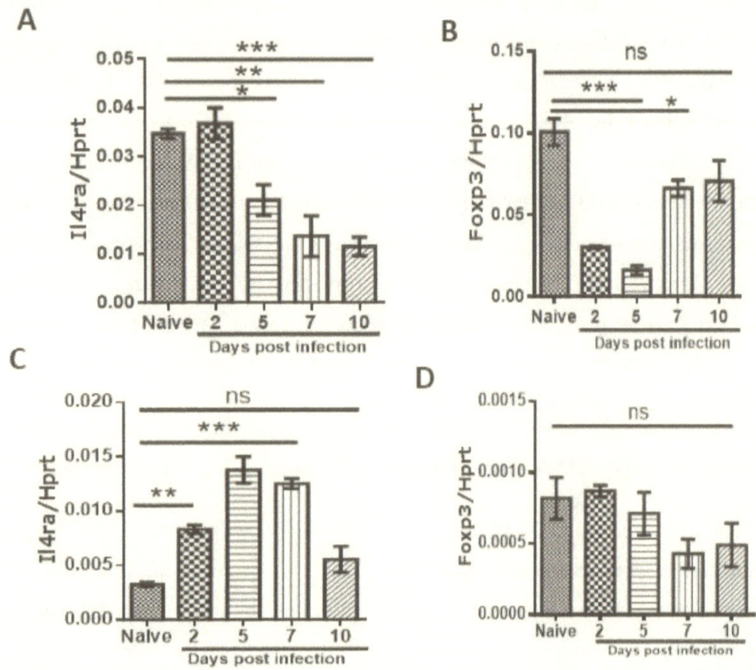

Figure 3. 1 mRNA expression of Il4rα and Foxp3 in spleen and liver of Lm infected mice: Mice were infected via an intraperitoneal route with $2x10^4$ CFU *Lm*. At the indicated days, mice were sacrificed to measure (A) Il4rα (B) Foxp3 mRNA levels from the spleen and (C) Il4rα and (D) Foxp3 in the liver. Data is normalized to Hprt housekeeping gene. Data represented as mean ± SEM of n=3 mice/time-point analysed by two-tailed, unpaired. Student t-test (*p<0.05, **p<0.01, ***p<0.001).

3.1.3 The IL-4Rα expression on Foxp3 T reg dynamics alters over the course of infection in Foxp3[cre]IL-4Rα[-/lox] mice during *Lm* infection.

We followed up the differences observed in IL-4Rα (Figure 1.1) *in vivo,* in mice lacking IL-4Rα specifically on Foxp3 T reg. Mice were infected with *Lm* with a sublethal dose of 2×10^4 *Lm*/200µl and sacrificed 3 and 7 days post-infection. Spleen and liver tissue were harvested to generate single-cell suspensions to determine the expression of IL-4Rα on Foxp3 T regs by flow cytometry. We found a significant reduction of IL-4Rα protein levels at 3 and 7dpi (Figure 3.2A & C) both in the spleen and the liver in Foxp3[cre]IL-4Rα[-/lox] animals relative to the littermate control, confirming a cell-specific deletion of the receptor on Foxp3 T regs in both organs during the course of the infection, as expected, not to the levels in global IL-4Rα knockouts. The characterization of Foxp3^{cre}IL-4Rα$^{-/lox}$ mice had been described by our group previously and there were not any irregularities reported in this mouse at (Aziz *et al.* 2018).

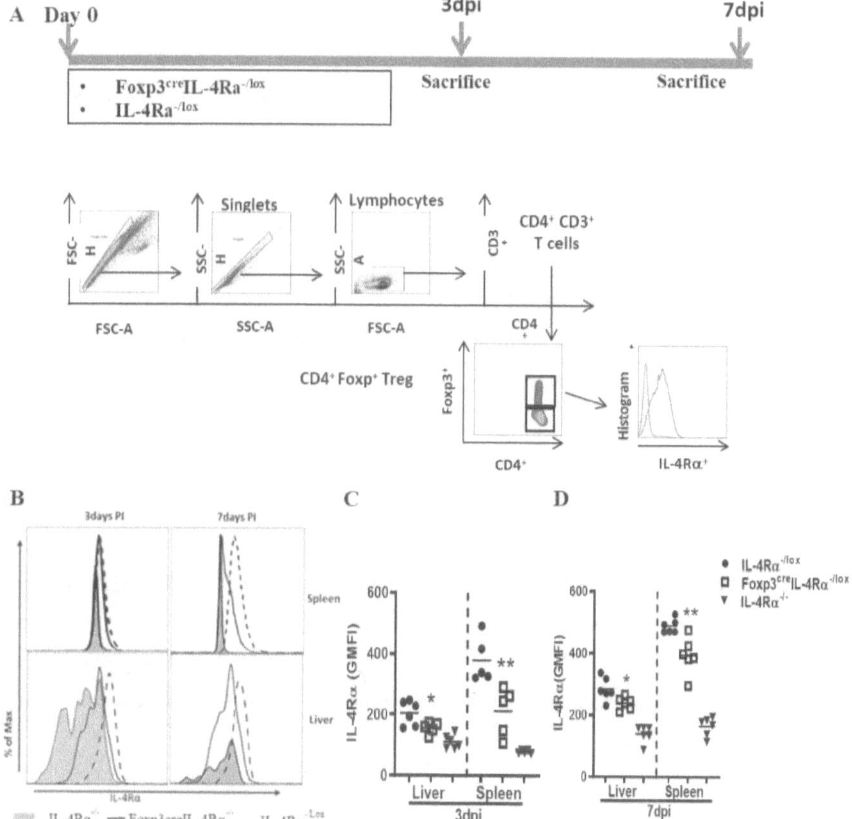

Figure 3.2 Confirmation of IL-4Rα knockdown in Foxp3 T cells during *Lm* infection. Mice were infected with low dose *Lm* 2×10^4 *Lm*/200μl, single-cell suspension from liver and spleen was generated and cells were analysed by flow cytometry to determine IL-4Rα expression on Foxp3 T regs (A) Diagramatic representation of *Lm* primary infection and gating strategy (B) Histogram representation from IL-4Rα$^{-/-}$ (grey tinted), Foxp3^{cre}IL-4Rα$^{-/lox}$ (solid line) and IL-4Rα$^{-/lox}$ (dashed line) tissues (C) IL-4Rα geometric mean fluorescence intensity (GMFI) quantification on spleen and liver at 3dpi and (D) 7dpi. Error bars denote mean ± SEM. Data shown are representative of 2 independent experiments. *n* = 5–7 mice/group. * $P < 0.05$, ** $P < 0.001$, *** $P < 0.0001$; Student's t-test.

3.14 Effect of IL-4Rα impairment on the functionality of Foxp3 T reg during *Lm* infection.

To assess whether the loss of IL-4Rα on Foxp3 T reg affected the quality of T regulatory cells (CD4$^+$ Foxp3), we use the expression of Foxp3 quantity (%) during infection by checking the expression of Foxp3$^+$GMFI by flow cytometry during *Lm* infection at 3 and 7 days in the spleen and liver. During shistosomaisis infection, STAT-6 phosphorylation in Foxp3^{cre}IL-4Rα$^{-/lox}$ mice was significantly reduced compared to IL-4Rα$^{-/lox}$ mice upon rIL-4 stimulation. Indicating the role of IL-4Rα in the stability of T regs during infection (Aziz *et al.* 2018). However, at a steady-state, the quality of the Foxp3 T reg population was not affected by the loss of the receptor. *In vitro* polarization experiments of sorted CD4$^+$CD25$^-$ cells by anti-CD3, anti-CD28 and TGF-β stimulation from Foxp3^{cre}IL-4Rα$^{-/lox}$ mouse showed a higher rate of conversion to CD4$^+$CD25$^+$ Foxp3 T cells (induced Treg cells) compared to littermate controls; however lower proliferative capacity.(Aziz *et al.* 2018) In infectious settings with *Schistosoma mansoni*, there was a significant decrease in the expression of Foxp3 on CD4 T cells and consequently an impaired accumulation of Foxp3 Treg cells at peripheral tissues (Aziz *et al.* 2018). Similarly, in *Lm* infection, there was a significant decrease in the expression of Foxp3 at 3dpi (Figure 3.3 A) and 7dpi (Figure 3B) in the spleen, but not in the liver tissue. This suggests that though the Foxp3 T regs population is not affected by the loss of IL-4Rα at a steady-state, during infection settings the quality and possible the functionality of Foxp3 T regs are affected. We did not observe much differences in the liver, probably due to insufficient deletion of IL-4Rα on T regs cells in the liver (Figure 3.3 A and B) or not as much T regs cells as in the spleen.

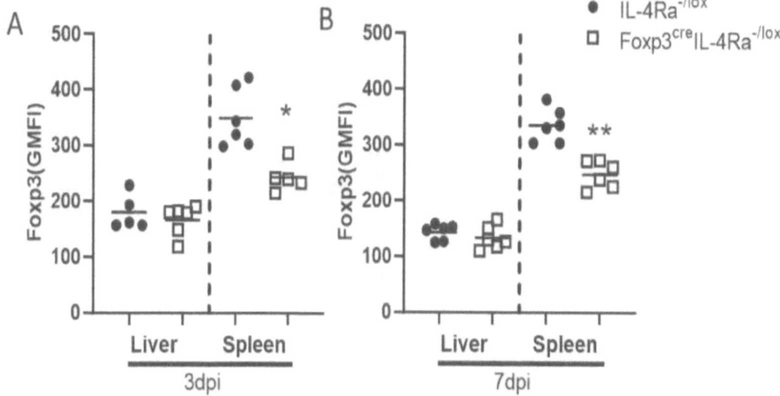

Figure 3.3 Functional decrease of Foxp3 in Foxp3^{cre}IL-4Rα$^{-/lox}$ mice in the spleen during *Lm* infection: Mice were infected with *Lm* via intraperitoneal injection with a sub-lethal dose of 2×10^4 CFU/200µl, mice were sacrificed at 3 and 7dpi and the expression Foxp3 on CD4$^+$ T cells are evaluated by flow cytometry. Foxp3 GMFI expression liver and spleen at (A) 3dpi and (B) 7dpi. Data are shown as mean ± SEM representative of three independent experiments, *, $p<0.05$, ** $p<0.01$. Student's t-test.

3.1.5 Foxp3^{cre}IL-4Rα$^{-/lox}$ mice survive better than their litter during *Lm* infection

With the quality of Foxp3 T regs being affected, we aim to understand the affect on survival and bacterial burden as a consequence of absence IL-4Rα on Foxp3 T reg during *Lm* infection. We infected a lethal dose (LD$_{50}$) of *Lm* (2×10^5 *Lm* CFU/mouse) intraperitoneally to Foxp3^{cre}IL-4Rα$^{-/lox}$ mice and littermate control (IL-4Rα$^{-/lox}$) animals. Higher mortality was observed in control littermate relative to Foxp3^{cre}IL-4Rα$^{-/lox}$ mice (Figure 3. 4A). This reveals a possible role IL-4Rα on Foxp3 during *Lm* infection possible as a consequence of reduced functional Foxp3 as observed in Figure 3.3. To better understand the survival of the Foxp3^{cre}IL-4Rα$^{-/lox}$ mice, we infected mice with a sublethal dose of *Lm* (2×10^4 Lm CFU/mouse) for time-kinetic experiments. At 3dpi and 7dpi, mice displayed a significantly reduced spleen bacterial burden (Figure 3.4B), but liver burdens were unaffected (Figure 3.4C). This suggests there is a tissue compartmentalized role of IL-4Rα on Foxp3 T reg during primary *Lm* infection.

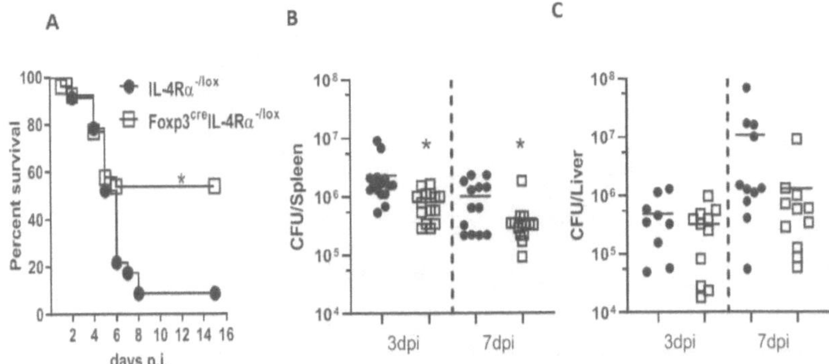

Figure 3.4 IL-4Rα deletion on Foxp3 T reg renders mice resistant to *Lm* infection. Mice were infected with *Lm* to evaluate survival and bacterial burden (A) Survival curve of Foxp3^{cre}IL-4Rα$^{-/lox}$ and littermate control (n=8-10 mice/group) following infection with a sub-lethal dose of 2x10^4 CFU/200μl *Lm*. Statistical significance determined by two-tailed Mantel-Cox test (p= 0.0123) (B) Spleen and (C) liver bacterial burden was determined at 3- and 7-days post-infection following infection with 2x10^4 CFU (n=10-15mice/group). Error bars denote mean ± mean and representative of two experiments (A) or pooled from four independent experiments (B-C). Data analysied by two-tailed unpaired Student's t-test, unpaired.*, P < 0.05; **, P < 0.01; ***, P < 0.001

3.1.6 Absence of IL-4Rα on Foxp3 T reg results in the reduced pathology and lesion size in liver and spleen during *Lm* infection

Since FoxP3^{cre}IL-4Rα$^{-/lox}$ mice survive better to *Lm* in the mortality study (Figure 3.4A), we performed hematoxylin and eosin staining (H&E) to evaluate histopathology of the spleen and liver during *Lm* infection as described above. At 3 and 7 days post-infection, Foxp3^{cre}IL-4Rα$^{-/lox}$ mice displayed smaller lesion size measured by atrophic white splenic pulp compared to their littermate control (Figure 3.5A). Similarly, in the liver, we observed decreased lession size in Foxp3^{cre}IL-4Rα$^{-/lox}$ mice when compared to littermate control (IL-4Rα$^{-/lox}$) mice (Figure 3.5B). This suggests that deletion of IL-4Rα on T regulatory cells decreased cellular infiltration into the tissues and consequently the lesion sizes.

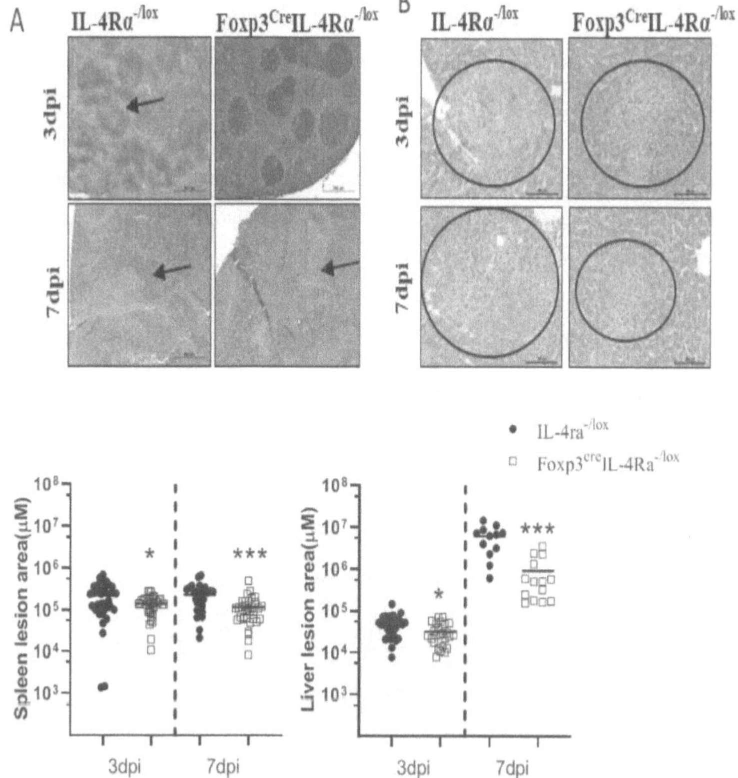

Figure 3.5 Decreased tissue pathology in Foxp3^{cre}IL-4Rα$^{-/lox}$ mice during *Lm* infection in peripheral organs. Foxp3^{cre}IL-4Rα$^{-/lox}$ and littermate control mice were intra-peritoneally infected with 2×10^4 *Lm*/200μl. At 3 dpi and 7dpi spleen and liver, tissues were formalin-fixed and stained with H&E for histopathology. Three cuts 30μm apart per histology sections were analysed (30μm apart, scale bar =100μm) (A) Diagrammatic representation of spleen with arrows showing white pulp atrophy. (magnification ×200, circled areas indicates cellular infiltration). (B) Diagrammatic representation of cellular infiltration into liver tissue (C) Quantification of splenic atrophic areas; (D) quantification of liver lesion size. Results are representative of three independent experiments with 6 to 8 mice/group. Data are expressed as mean ± mean, two-tailed unpaired Student t test . $P > 0.05$; * $P < 0.05$, ** $P < 0.001$, *** $P < 0.0001$.

3.1.7 Liver cytokine reponses in Foxp3^{cre}IL-4Rα$^{-/lox}$ mice during *Lm*

To understand the underlying cause of Foxp3^{cre}IL-4Rα$^{-/lox}$ survival benefit (Figure 3.4A) and improved histopathology (Figure 3.5B), we performed cytokine ELISA on liver homogenates at 3 and 7 days post-infection. At 3 days post-infection, there was a significant decrease in pro-inflammatory cytokines; IFN-γ, IL-12p40, and IL-6, however, TGF-β, TNF, IL-4 and IL-10 levels remained unaffected (Figure 3.6A). In contrast at 7 days post-infection, there was a significant increase in TNF, IL-10 and IL-4, suggesting a dampening effect in the absence of IL-4Rα on Foxp3 T regs; however, there were no differences in IL-17, IFN-γ, TGF-β, IL-12p40 and IL-6 at this time-point (Figure 3.6B). Decreased pro-inflammatory cytokines also account for reduced tissue damage at the liver.

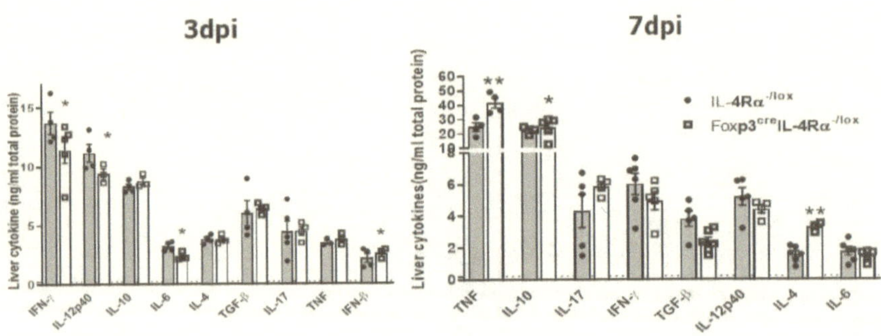

Figure 3.6 Lack of IL-4Rα expression on Foxp3 T reg cells impairs hepatic cytokines during *Lm* infection. Mice were infected intra peritoneally with $2×10^4$ *Lm* and sacrificed 3dpi and 7dpi and cytokines ELISAs performed on liver homogenates at (A) 3dpi and (B) 7dpi. Error bars denote mean ± SEM. Data shown are representative of one of three independent experiments with a sample size of n = 6–8 mice per group and analysed by two-tailed, unpaired, Student's t-test. *p < 0.05, **p < 0.01, and ***p < 0.001

3.1.8 *Ex vivo* stimulation of splenocytes show a proinflammatory cytokine profile in mice lacking IL-4Rα on Foxp3 T regs during *Lm* infection

We next examined the spleen cytokine profile following restimulation with either heat-killed *Lm* (HLKM) or anti-CD3 or left unstimulated (Figure 3.7A-E). At 3dpi, there were no major differences in the cytokine profiles in IFN-γ, IL-10, and TNF (Figure 3A-C). At 7dpi, there was a significant increase in IFN-γ and IL-10 upon anti-CD3 stimulation (Figure 3.7D-E). This modest increase in IFN-γ likely contributed in observed decreased bacterial burdens can be an indicator of bacterial clearance since IFN-γ increase plays a cricial role in the clearance of *Lm* clearance during infection (Buchmeier & Schreiber 1985).

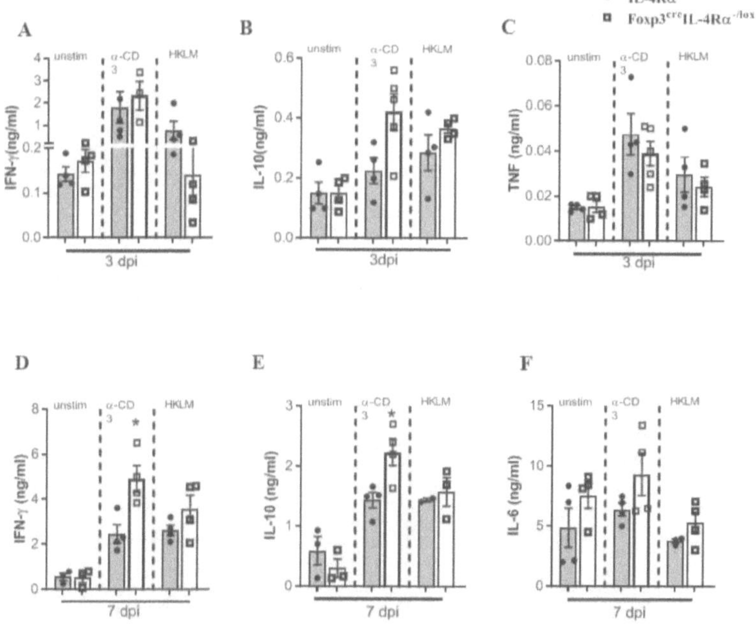

Figure 3.7 Pro-inflammatory cytokines are enhanced in Foxp3^{cre}IL-4Rα$^{-/lox}$ mice during *Lm* infection. Spleen cells were re-stimulated with α-CD3 and heat-killed *Lm* (HKLM) or left unstimulated for 72 hours, after which cytokines were measured in the supernatants by ELISA at 3dpi (A) IFN-γ (B) IL-10 (C) TNF and at 7dpi (D) IFN-γ (E) IL-10 (F) IL-6. Data is representative of two individual experiments with mean values ± SEM. Statistical analysis was performed, by two-tailed unpaired Student t-test,(*, p<0.05, **, p<0.01)

3.1.9 Pro-inflammatory cytokines are enhanced in the sera of Foxp3^{cre}IL-4Rα$^{-/lox}$ mice during *Lm* infection

Since we observed an increase in IFN-γ secretion upon splenocyte restimulation, we sought to investigate whther serum cytokines were affected differentially in Foxp3^{cre}IL-4Rα$^{-/lox}$ mice during *Lm* infection with sub-lethal dose. There was a significant increase in IL-1β (Figure 3.8A), increase in IL-12p70 (Figure 3.8B), increase in IFN-γ (Figure 3.8C) and increase in

TGF-β (Figure 3.8F) at 7dpi for Foxp3^{cre}IL-4Rα$^{-/lox}$ mice. There was no change in TNF (Figure 3.8E) and a decrease in IL-1β and IL-1α at 3dpi respectively (Figure 3.8 A&D). An increase in pro-inflmammtory cytokines in serum including IFN-γ suggests an important role of IL-4Rα signalling on Foxp3 in controlling dissemination from the organs in later stages of infection.

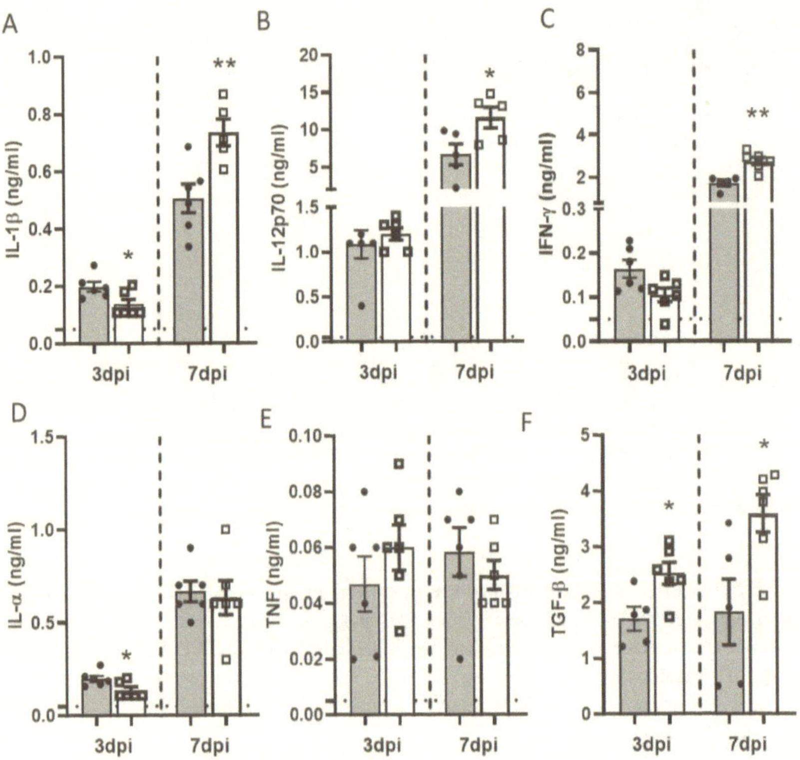

Figure 3.8 Increased serum cytokine secretion in Foxp3^{cre}IL-4Rα$^{-/lox}$ mice. Mice were infected with a sublethal dose *Lm* (2×10^4 CFU) Cytokine concentrations were measured in the serum by ELISA at 3 and 7 dpi (A) IL-1β, (B) IL-12p70 (C) IFN-γ, (D) IL-1α, (E), TNF and (F), TGF-β. Data is representative of two individual experiments with mean ± SEM. Grey bars representing IL-4Rα$^{-/Lox}$, white bars Foxp3^{cre}IL-4Rα$^{-/lox}$ mice. Statistical analysis was performed by two-tailed unpaired Student t-test. (*, $p \leq 0.05$, **, $p \leq 0.01$)

3.1.10 Absence of IL-4Rα signalling on Foxp3[cre]IL-4Rα[-/lox] mice alter cell numbers and myeloid population during *Lm* infection

To better understand which cell population were involved for the augmented infiltration (Figure 3.5 A-D), animals were infected with a sub lethal dose of *Lm* and sacrificed at 3 and 7dpi. Single-cell suspensions were prepared from the liver and spleen and analysed for the myeloid cell populations. We first evaluated the total cell numbers in the spleen and liver. There was a significant increase in total cell numbers cell numbers in the Foxp3[cre]IL-4Rα[-/lox] mice compared to littermate controls in the spleen at 3 and 7 dpi (Figure 3.9A) but no significant differences at the liver (Figure 3.9B). There was a significant increase of macrophage population in the Foxp3[cre]IL-4Rα[-/lox] mice at 7dpi (Figure 3.9 C) and a significant increase of DCs at 3 dpi (Figure 3.9 D) in the spleen. In addition, an increase of neutrophils at both 3 and 7 dpi in the Foxp3[cre]IL-4Rα[-/lox] mice was observed. There was a decreased number of macrophages in the liver at both time points. (Figure 3.9 F) and a decrease in neutrophils at 7 dpi (Figure 3.9 H). There were no differences in DCs in the liver at both time points (Figure 3.9 G). An increase in neutrophil is known to control *Lm* during the early stages of the disease which can explain decreased splenic bacterial burden in the Foxp3[cre]IL-4Rα[-/lox] mice (Witter *et al.* 2016). This shows that the recruitment of infiltrating populations varied between the spleen and liver during *Lm* infection in Foxp3[cre]IL-4Rα[-/lox] mice.

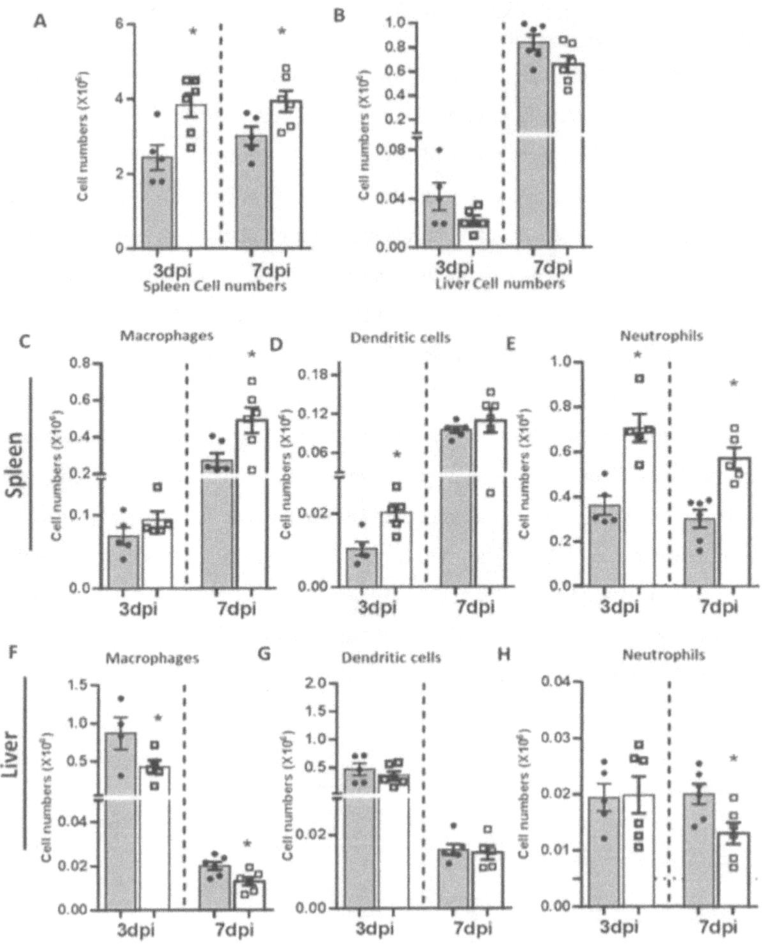

Figure 3.9 Foxp3^{cre}IL-4Rα^{-/lox} mice showed increased total cell numbers and myeloid cell population in the spleen during *Lm*. Mice were intraperitoneally infected with *Lm*, total cell counts were counted by Trypan Blue exclusion assay. Extracellular staining was performed on macrophages, dendritic cells, and neutrophils at 3 and 7dpi. (A) Spleen total cell counts, (B) total cell count numbers in the liver. Spleen (C) macrophage, (D) DC, (E) neutrophil, and liver (F) monocyte-derived macrophage, (G) DC and (H) neutrophil counts are shown. Data is representative of two experiments. Grey bars representing IL-4Rα^{-/Lox}, white bars representing Foxp3^{cre}IL-4Rα^{-/lox} mice. All data are shown as mean ± SEM and are representative of two independents experiments, compared to control. Data is analysed by a two-tailed unpaired Student t-test. * $P < 0.05$, ** $P < 0.01$

3.1.11 Absence IL-4Rα signalling on Foxp3[cre]IL-4Rα [-/lox] mice on other lymphoid cells during *Lm* infection

Cytokine secretion during infection affect T cells and their surrounding cells. We evaluated T cells since they play an important role during *Lm* infection (Shedlock *et al.* 2003; Pamer 2004; Graw *et al.* 2012). We showed that loss of IL-4Rα signalling on Foxp3 [cre]IL-4Rα [-/lox] mice affected the secretion of pro-inflammatory cytokines (Figures 3.6, 3.7 & 3.8), improved histopathology (Figure 3.5) and enhanced survival (Figure 3.4). We investigated T cell population to evaluate the effect on lymphocyte populations (CD4[+]T cell and CD8[+]T cell) in the liver and spleen at 3 and 7dpi. CD4[+] T cell at the spleen and liver was similar for both groups except there was a slight decrease in CD4[+] T cells at 7dpi in the liver at 7dpi (Figure 3.10A and C). There was a significant increase of CD8[+] T cell population in the spleen (Figure 3.10B) whilst it remained unaffected in the liver (Figure 3.10B and D). Since CD8[+] T cells are very important for *Lm* clearance (Tvinnereim *et al.* 2002; Zaiss *et al.* 2008) their increased numbers in Foxp3[cre]IL-4Rα [-/lox] mice are quite notable and we further analysed these cells to understand the secretion of other intracellular cytokines and granzyme-B produced mainly by CD8[+] cytotoxic T cells.

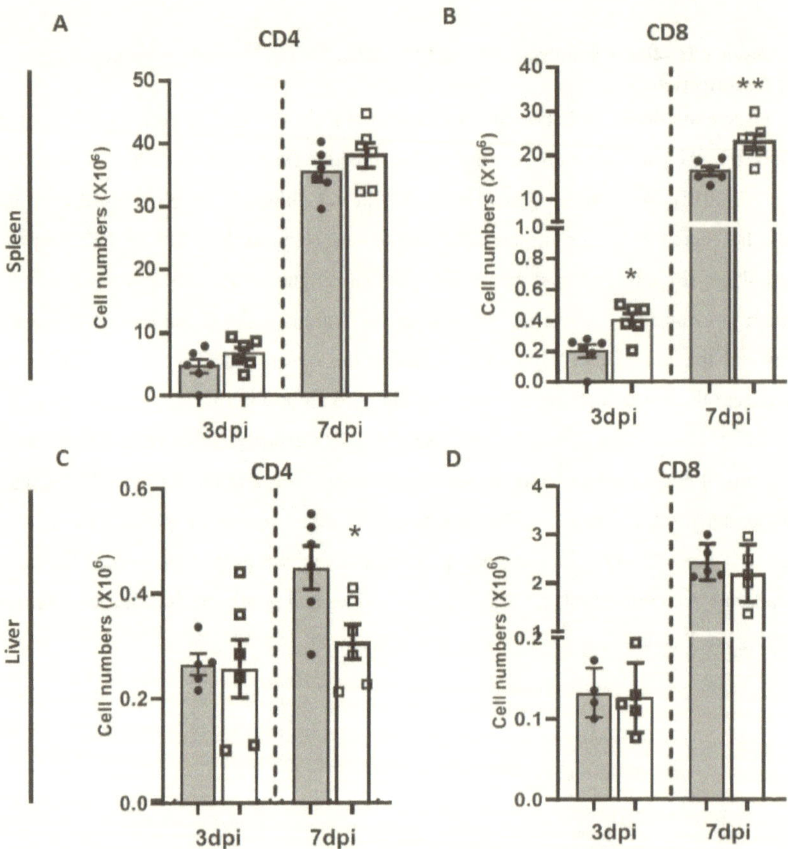

Figure 3.10 CD4/CD8 T cells population during _Lm_ infection of Foxp3^{cre}IL-4Rα$^{-/lox}$ mice:. Mice were infected with $2x10^4$ CFU via intraperitoneal injection. Single cell suspensions of total splenic and liver cells were prepared and stained for (A) CD4 spleen cells, (B) CD8 spleen cells, (C) CD4 liver cells, (D) CD8 liver cells and acquired on BD Fortessa. Grey bars representing IL-4Rα$^{-/Lox}$, white bars representing Foxp3^{cre}IL-4Rα$^{-/lox}$ mice. Data are presented as mean ± SEM of n=6-8 mice/time point from three independent experiments and analysed by two-tailed unpaired Student t-test *p<0.05, **p<0.01

3.1.12 Ex-vivo T cell cytokine responses in Foxp3^{cre}IL-4Rα$^{-/lox}$ mice during *Lm* infection

With an increased IFN-γ released by splenocytes (Figure 3.7D), serum (Figure 3.8C), and increased CD8$^+$ T cell numbers at 7dpi (Figure 3.10B); we sought to understand the underlying mechanism in the spleen at 7dpi. We infected mice with 2×10^4 CFUs low dose *Lm* and sacrificed at 7dpi. Taking into consideration that CD8$^+$ cytotoxic T cell is one of the predominant cellular population that kills *Lm* (Harty & Badovinac 2002); we re-stimulated cells with heat-killed *Lm* (HKLM), PMA/ionomycin or left unstimulated to perform intracellular cytokine staining for IFN-γ, IL-2, IL-17, TNF and granzyme B. In unstimulated cells, there was a significant increase in CD4$^+$ T producing IFN-γ and IL-2 in Foxp3^{cre}IL-4Rα$^{-/lox}$ mice (Figure 3.11A) but not in CD8$^+$ T cells. Stimulation with HKLM also led to increases in IL-2 but not in IFN-γ, IL-17 and TNF in both in the CD4$^+$ and CD8$^+$ T cells. (Figure 3.11B). Moreover, stimulation with PMA/ionomycin led to a significant increase in the production of IFN-γ and IL-2 but not in IL-17 and TNF levels in both CD4 and CD8 T cells of Foxp3^{cre}IL-4Rα$^{-/lox}$ mice (Figure 3.11C). Granzyme B is an important *Listeria monocytogenes* host killing protease produced by cytotoxic cells, thus we checked if the deletion of IL-4Rα signalling of T regs affected the ability of CD4$^+$ T cells and CD8$^+$ T cells to produced granzyme B. Granzyme B is critical for the killing of *Listeria monocytogenes* (Kaufmann 1993). In addition to CD8+ T cells activated CD4 T cells are also known to produce granzyme B (Takeuchi & Saito 2017). We observed a significant increase in the production of granzyme B production in both CD4$^+$ T cell and CD8$^+$ T cells in Foxp3^{cre}IL-4Rα$^{-/lox}$ mice. (Figure 3.11D and E). These results suggest abrogation of IL-4Rα on Foxp3 T reg might play a role in a shift to a Th1 and cytotoxic phenotype.

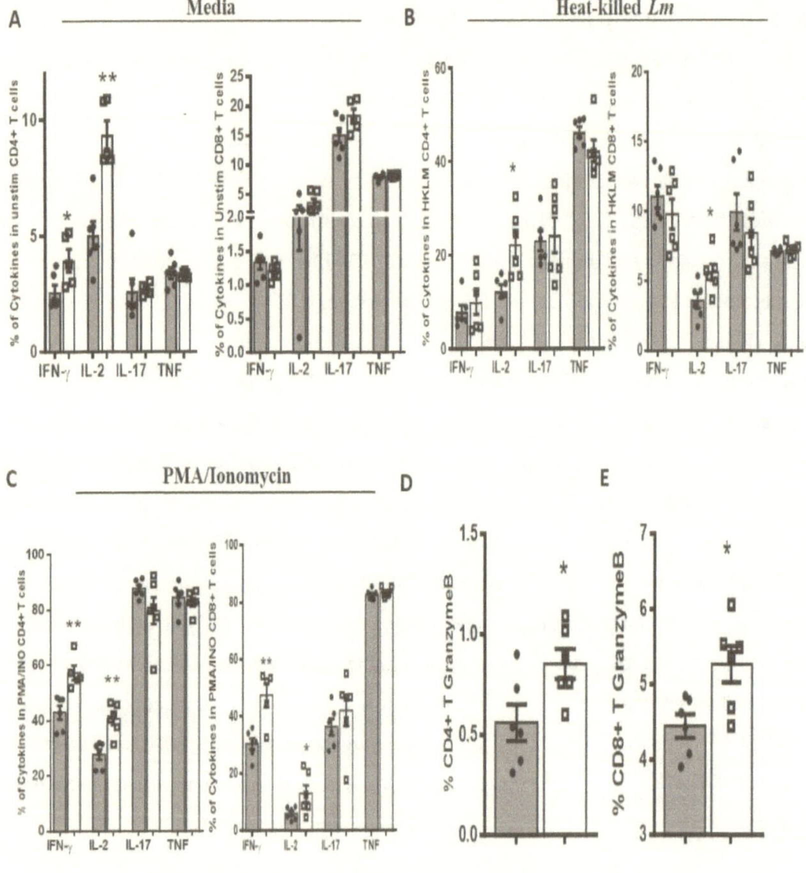

Figure 3.11 Intracellular cytokine profile in splenic T cells during *Lm* infection. Animals were intraperitoneally infected with 2x10^4 *Lm*. Single cell suspension was prepared and 2 million cells were then seeded to either stimulate cells in (A) media (B) heat-killed *Lm* and (C) PMA(20ng/ml)/ionomycin(1µg/ml) (D) Splenic CD4 T cell GranzymeB (E) Splenic CD8 T cell GranzymeB for 6 hours followed by monensin 200µM blockage to perform intracellular cytokine staining and acquired on the Fortessa. Grey bars representing IL-4Rα$^{-/Lox}$, white bars representing Foxp3^{cre}IL-4Rα$^{-/lox}$ mice. Data represented as mean ± SEM of n=6 mice/time point from three independent experiments and analysed by two-tailed unpaired Student t-test (*p<0.05, **p<0.01)

3.1.13 Effector CD4$^+$ T cell memory responses in Foxp3^{cre}IL-4Rα $^{-/lox}$ mice are enhanced during *Lm* infection

After infection with *Lm*, CD4$^+$T cells are activated. Considering that, we noticed a continuous increase in IFN-γ cytokine in the splenic cells (Figure 3.7D), serum (Figure 3.8C) and in *ex vivo* stimulated splenic cells (Figure 3.11). We next asked if these cells had augmented effector phenotype in the Foxp3^{cre}IL-4Rα$^{-/lox}$ mice at 7 days post-infection. Foxp3^{cre}IL-4Rα$^{-/lox}$ mice had significantly higher effector/effector memory phenotype (CD44^{high}CD62L^{low}) compared to littermate controls (Figure 3.12). This high effector phenotype can possibly explain the IFN-γ production; a key Th1 response cytokine. Collectively, this data suggests that upon deletion of IL-4Rα on Foxp3^{cre}IL-4Rα$^{-/lox}$ mice, an augmented effector T cell memory phenotype is acquired that leads to the production of IFN-γ and IL-2 cytokines. Also, CD4$^+$ T cells and CD8$^+$T cells produced increased granzyme B in Foxp3^{cre}IL-4Rα$^{-/lox}$ mice.

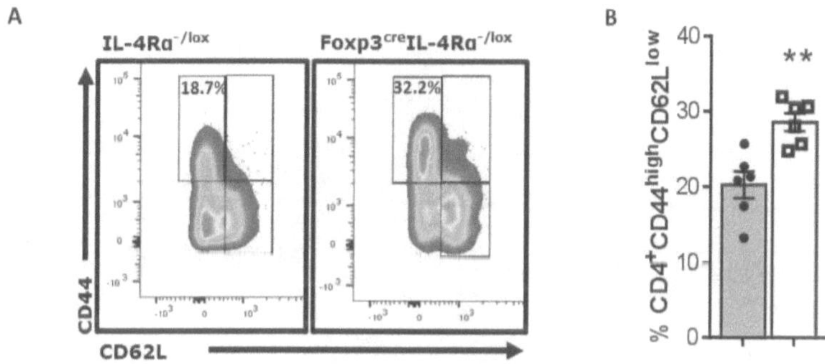

Figure 3.12 Abrogation of IL-4Rα expression on Foxp3 cells enhance CD4 T cell effector function. Mice were infected with 2x10^4 CFU via intraperitoneal injection. A single-cell suspension of total splenic cells analysed to determine effector T cell proportion by flow cytometry. (A) Diagrammatic representation of the effector population pre-gated on CD4 cells. (B) Quantification (%) of effector T cells. Grey bars representing IL-4Rα$^{-/Lox}$, white bars representing Foxp3^{cre}IL-4Rα$^{-/lox}$ mice. Data represented as mean ± SEM of n=6-8 mice/time point from three independent experiments and analysed by two-tailed, unpaired Student t-test (*p<0.05, **p<0.01).

3.1.14 Absence IL-4Rα expression on Foxp3 T reg cells enhance Tbet signature

In order to delineate the effector phenotype function coupled with IFN-γ production in serum and spleen; we checked the expression of transcriptional factor T-bet on T helper and cytotoxic T cells. The T-bet expression is known for the control of the Th1 phenotype and production of cytokines like IFN-γ, IL-2, and TNF (Szabo *et al.* 2000). Remarkably, the absence of IL-4Rα on Foxp3 T reg cells resulted in a significant increase in the percentage of T-bet expression in both CD4$^+$ T cells and CD8$^+$ T cells upon *Lm* infection at 7dpi (Figure 3.13A-D). The T-bet transcriptional factor is known to promote the growth and differentiation of the Th1 subset while concomitantly blocking the other subsets (Seder & Paul 1994). However, we found no differences in GATA3 in Foxp3^{cre}IL-4Rα$^{-/lox}$ mice (Figure 3.13E and F). These results suggest that there is a shift towards a Th1 phenotype in the absence of IL-4Rα expression on Foxp3 T reg cells during *Lm* infection

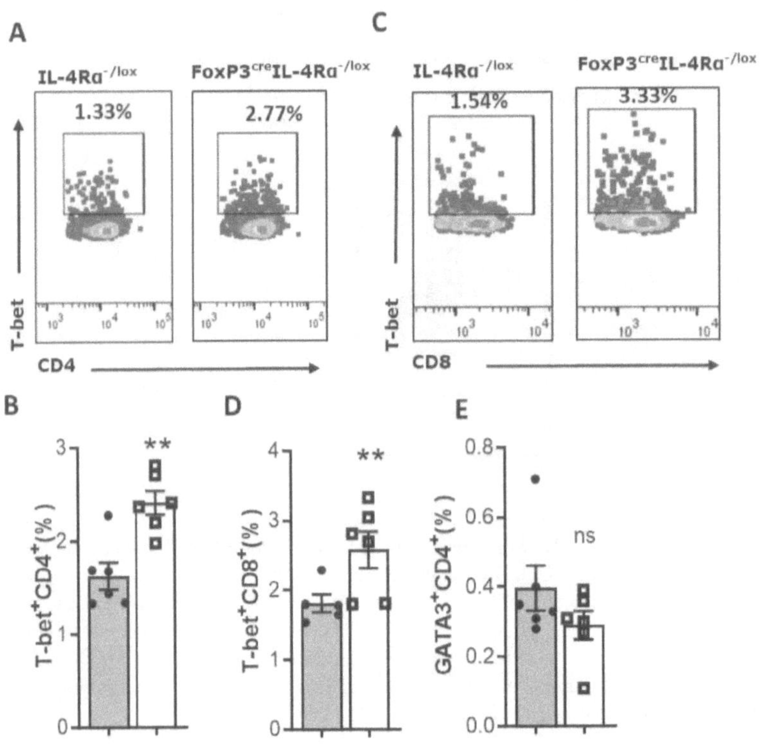

Figure 3.13 T-bet transcriptional factor expression is significantly enhanced in Foxp3^{cre}IL-4Rα $^{-/lox}$ mice during *Lm* infection. Mice were infected intraperitoneally with 2 x 10^4 *Lm*. A single-cell suspension of total splenic cells was stained for intranuclear transcriptional factors T-bet and GATA-3 from mice sacrificed at 7dpi (A) Representative flow cytometry plot of the frequency of T-bet$^+$ CD4$^+$ (C) T-bet$^+$ CD8$^+$, (B) quantification of T-bet$^+$ CD4$^+$ and (D) T-bet$^+$ CD4$^+$ populations. (E) frequency of GATA-3$^+$CD4$^+$ cells. Grey bars representing IL-4Rα$^{-/Lox}$ mice while white bars Foxp3^{cre}IL-4Rα$^{-/lox}$ mice. Data shown are representative of two independent experiments (*p<0.05, **p<0.01) analysed by two-tailed unpaired Student t-test

3.1.15 Abrogated IL-4Rα-mediated signalling on Foxp3 T reg cells leads to expansion and survival of CD8$^+$ T cells during *Lm* infection.

To better understand the histopathological destruction of white splenic pulp in the littermate control compared to Foxp3^{cre}IL-4Rα$^{-/lox}$ at 7 dpi, we checked activated caspase 3 expression which is a marker of apoptosis, the physiological process in the elimination of cells. We also assessed the anti-apoptotic B cells lymphoma-2 (Bcl-2) expression since it is known to inhibit apoptosis (Bissonnette *et al.* 1992). It has been reported that infection with *Lm* causes the destruction of the white pulp by apoptosis *in vitro* and *in vivo* (Carrero *et al.* 2004). Therefore, we assessed the deletion of IL-4Rα deletion on T regs and the effect on apoptosis and survival of CD8$^+$ T cells. Also, we asked if the absence of IL-4Rα on T reg could lead to more expansion and survival of these CD8$^+$ T cells as observed in Figure 3.10B. We hypothesized this based on reduced Foxp3 T reg population in the IL-4Rα deficient T reg mice (Figure 3.3) and might affect the effect the T reg/effector balance. The presence of Bcl-2 and Ki-67 markers are indicators of cell proliferation and nuclear protein activity during cell division. We investigated CD8/CD4 T cell proliferation. We observed significant increase in CD8$^+$Ki-67$^+$ (Figure 3.14A&B) and CD8$^+$BCL-2$^+$ Caspase3$^+$ (Figure 3.14C) in Foxp3^{cre}IL-4Rα$^{-/lox}$ mice. However, no differences in CD4$^+$Ki-67$^+$ (Figure 3.14F), CD4$^+$BCL-2$^+$ (Figure 3.14F) and CD4$^+$Caspase3$^+$ (Figure 3.14G). Following expansion, most CD8 T cells die after infection, with lesser memory population that is capable of surviving and offering long lasting protection during the subsequent challenge from the same antigen (D'Cruz *et al.* 2009). These results suggest in the absence of IL-4Rα on Foxp3 T regs, CD8 T cells expand, with decreased apoptosis and better survival. We did not, however, check on long term memory and survival at later time point.

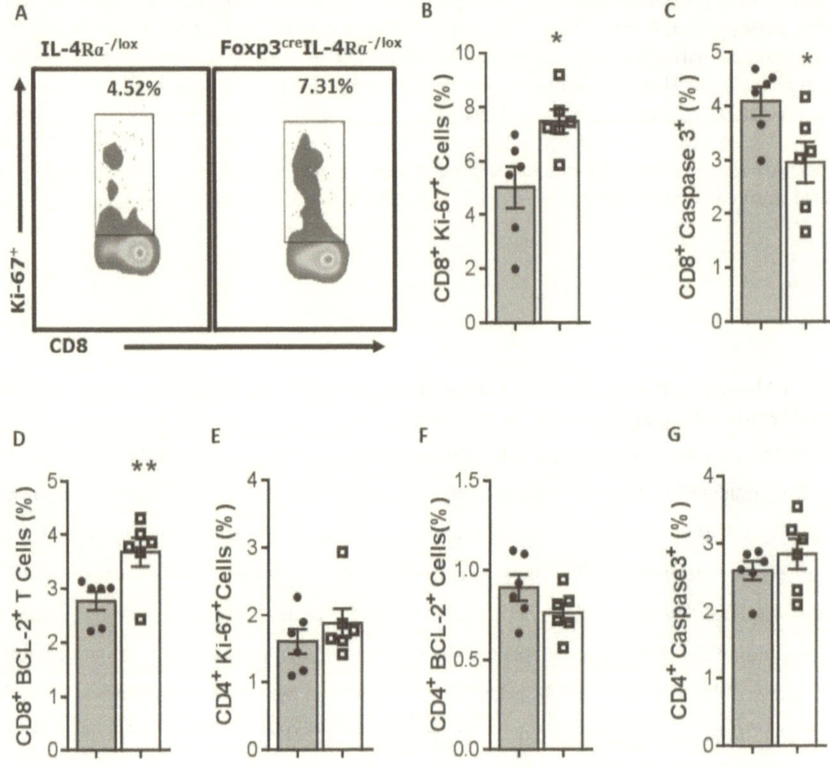

Figure 3.14 CD8$^+$ T cells significantly expand in the spleen of Foxp3^{cre}IL-4Rα$^{-/lox}$ mice during *Lm* infection: Mice were infected intraperitoneally with low dose *Lm* (2x4^{10}CFU/mouse). A single-cell suspension of total splenic cells was stained for BCL-2 and Ki-67 protein in CD8/CD4 T cells 7dpi. (A) Frequency of CD8$^+$Ki-67$^+$ (B) quantification of CD8$^+$Ki-67$^+$ (C) CD8$^+$Caspase3$^+$ T cells (D) CD8$^+$BCL-2$^+$ T cell (E) CD4$^+$Ki-67$^+$ T cells (F) CD4$^+$BCL-2$^+$ T cells and (G) CD4$^+$Caspase3$^+$ T cells. Grey bars representing IL-4Rα$^{-/Lox}$ mice while white bars Foxp3^{cre}IL-4Rα$^{-/lox}$ mice Data represented as mean ± SEM of n=6-8 mice/time point from two independent experiments and analysed by two-tailed unpaired Student t-test (*p<0.05, **p<0.01)

3.1.16 A shift towards Th1-type immune responses in Foxp3^{cre}IL-4R$\alpha^{-/lox}$ T cells during *ex vivo* stimulation

In order to determine whether the increased protection observed in Foxp3^{cre}IL-4R$\alpha^{-/lox}$ mice during primary infection with *Lm* was accompanied by an altered immune response *ex vivo*, we examined cellular activation and cytokine responses by flow cytometry in a co-culture of bone marrow-derived macrophages (BMDM) and T cells from Foxp3^{cre}IL-4R$\alpha^{-/lox}$ mice and littermate controls. In naïve mice, CD4$^+$CD25$^+$ are widely used as a marker for T reg. The depletion of CD25$^+$ in naïve mice has been shown to develop autoimmunity similar to T regs (Foxp3) deficient (Setoguchi *et al.* 2005; Zelenay *et al.* 2005; Chai *et al.* 2008). We carried out co-culture experiment with a 1:1 ratio (macrophages: CD4$^+$CD25$^-$ T cells), 1:3 ratio (macrophages: CD4$^+$CD25$^-$ T cells) or 1:3:1 ratio (macrophages: CD4$^+$CD25$^-$ T cells: CD4$^+$CD25$^+$ T cells). Flow analysis revealed a decreased population of T reg (CD4$^+$Foxp3$^+$) in the Foxp3^{cre}IL-4R$\alpha^{-/lox}$ mice compared to the littermate control (Figure 3.15A). This was in line with *in vivo* results obtained in Figure 3.3 and the presence of CD4$^+$CD25$^+$ cells evidently increased the Foxp3 signature. We performed T cell effector functions on the various groups. In the group of ratios 1: 3, there was a significant increase in CD4 effector function in both groups evident of the addition of CD4$^+$CD25$^-$ effector cells. There were no differences between the T cells isolated from littermate control and Foxp3^{cre}IL-4R$\alpha^{-/lox}$ spleens. Upon the addition of CD4$^+$CD25$^+$ T cells (T regs), there was a suppression of the effector function (Figure 3.15B). There were no differences in central memory in the different subsets. The addition of T regs significantly suppressed central memory (Figure 3.15C). There was an increase in naïve T cells with the increased CD4 T effector cell ratios. Strikingly there was an increase naïve T cell phenotype in the Foxp3^{cre}IL-4R$\alpha^{-/lox}$ mice in the (1:3:1 ratio) group than littermate control (Figure 3.15D). There was a significantly increased proliferation of T cells from ratio 1:3 compared to ratio 1:1, proliferation was not affected by the addition of T regs (ratio 1:3:1). We did not observe differences between Foxp3^{cre}IL-4R$\alpha^{-/lox}$ mice and littermate controls within each group (Figure 3.15E). Consistent with *in vivo* results, where increased proliferation was observed only with CD8$^+$ T cells but not in CD4$^+$ T cell.

We further analysed the cytokines from supernatants and found IL-1β was significantly increased when T cells added to macrophage co-culture, most probably due to the activation of macrophages by IFN-γ. This was significantly reduced with the addition of T regs though no differences were found between the groups (Figure 3.15G). There were no differences in IFN-γ

secretion between T cells from the littermate controls and Foxp3^{cre}IL-4Rα$^{-/lox}$ (Figure 3.15H). IL-10 was secreted by macrophages and in the presence of T regs in a significant amount compared to groups with no T regs. Interestingly mice lacking IL-4Rα on T regs showed lesser secretion of IL-10 compared to the littermate control, suggesting compromised suppressive function (Figure 3.15I). Therefore, the absence of IL-4Rα on T regs (Figure 3.15D) led to significant increase in CD4 effector function during *Lm* infections in conformity with the *in vivo* results.

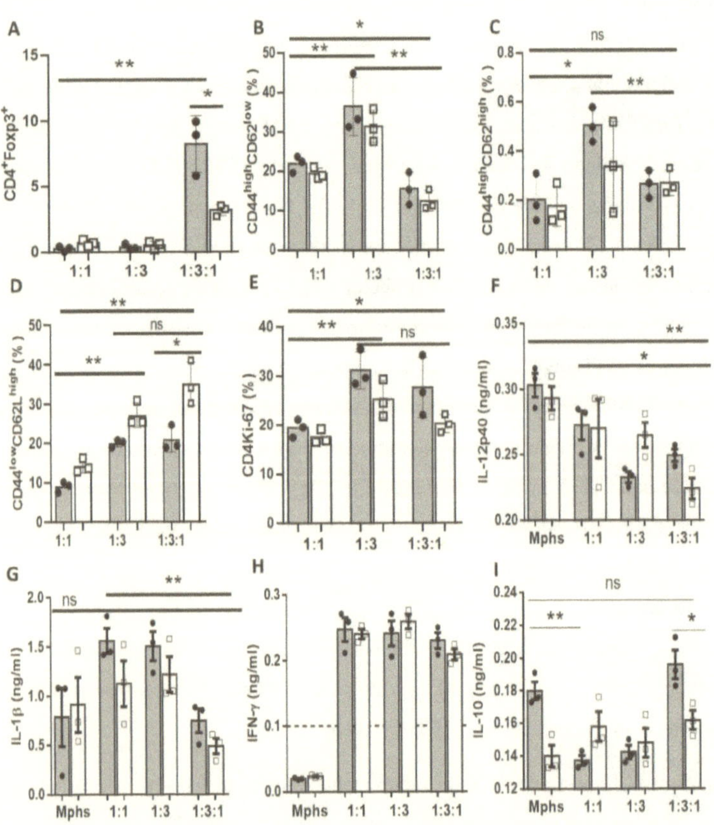

Figure 3.15 Decreased suppressive capacity of T regs from Foxp3^{cre}IL-4Rα^{-/lox} mice in vitro BMDMs were derived from IL-4Rα^{-/lox} mice, co-cultured with T cells (CD4$^+$CD25$^-$ or CD4$^+$CD25$^+$) from IL-4Rα^{-/lox} and Foxp3^{cre}IL-4Rα^{-/lox} mice after stimulation with HKLM (MOI 1:5) for 72 hours. (A) Percentages of CD4$^+$Foxp3$^+$ cells, (B) CD4 T effector memory, (C) central memory, (D) naïve T cells determined by flow cytometry. (E) Ki-67 T cell proliferation, (F) IL-12p40, (G) IL-1β, (H) IFN-γ, (I) IL-10 cytokines determined ELISA. A single experiment is shown with values ± SEM of triplicates 1:1 ratio represents (1-macrophages: 1-CD4$^+$CD25$^-$ T cells), 1:3 ratio (1-macrophages: 3-CD4$^+$CD25$^-$ T cells) 1:3:1 ratio (1-macrophages: 3-CD4$^+$CD25$^-$ T cells: 1-CD4$^+$CD25$^+$ T cells). Statistical analysis was performed using unpaired Student t-test (*, $p \leq 0.05$, **, $p \leq 0.01$ ***, $p \leq 0.001$).

3.1.17 IL-4Rα-mediated signalling on Foxp3 T reg cells is indispensable for secondary responses in *Lm* infection

To further understand the role of IL-4Rα signalling on T reg during long term memory after immunization, littermate controls and Foxp3^{cre}IL-4Rα^{-/lox} mice were immunized with 1×10^4 CFU/mouse and left for 30 days to permit complete bacterial clearance and acquire immunological memory (Figure 3.16A). Mice were re-challenged 30 days after with a lethal dose, 100 times the dose of the primary vaccination (1×10^6). Mice were monitored for mortality. In parallel, mice were sacrificed at two days post-infection to assess the spleen and liver burden. Increased mortality was observed in Foxp3^{cre}IL-4Rα^{-/lox} mice compared to their littermate control (Figure 3.16B). Strikingly, 50% of the control littermates survived after 15 days whereas all the Foxp3^{cre}IL-4Rα^{-/lox} mice died before day 6. Consistent with survival, Foxp3^{cre}IL-4Rα^{-/lox} mice had significantly increased bacterial burden both in the spleen and the liver (Figure 3.16B). Susceptibility to infection in Foxp3^{cre}IL-4Rα^{-/lox} mice was accompanied by a significant increase in spleen and liver lesions (Figure 3.16 C and D). To better understand why the Foxp3^{cre}IL-4Rα^{-/lox} mice were susceptible despite initial protection in the primary infection, we performed cytokine ELISA on the liver homogenates, intracellular flow cytometry for spleen cytokines. In the liver, there were significant increases in IFN-γ, TGF-β, IL-10 and IL-12p70 (Figure 3.16F) levels in Foxp3^{cre}IL-4Rα^{-/lox} mice. On the other hand, there was a slight decrease in IL-1α and IL-1β (Figure 3.16F) in mice lacking IL-4Rα specifically on Foxp3 T reg. IL-10 and TGF-β are well known immune-regulatory cytokines that act in to protect tissues and limit damages from excessive pro-inflammatory responses. However, excessive production can also inhibit the effector function of the pro-inflammatory cytokines. (Sanjabi *et al.* 2009; Barbosa *et al.* 2015). Paradoxically, there was a significant secretion of IFN-γ, and IL-12p70 pro-inflammatory cytokines. There were no significant differences in IL-4 secretion at the liver. These results suggest that pro-inflammatory cytokine secretion is sustained in Foxp3^{cre}IL-4Rα$^{-/lox}$ mice during a re-challenged that might likely contribute to tissue damage and therefore increased mortality. Single-cell CD4^{+} T cells staining revealed a significant increase in IL-4 and IL-10 and a decrease in IFN-γ in Foxp3^{cre}IL-4Rα$^{-/lox}$ mice. This suggests IL-4 and IL-10 might be inhibiting the IFN-γ which is necessary for *Lm* clearance, hence the observed increased bacterial burden in the spleen. (Figure 3.16G) This shows that intact IL-4Ra signalling is required to modulate host immune responses during secondary infection with *Lm*.

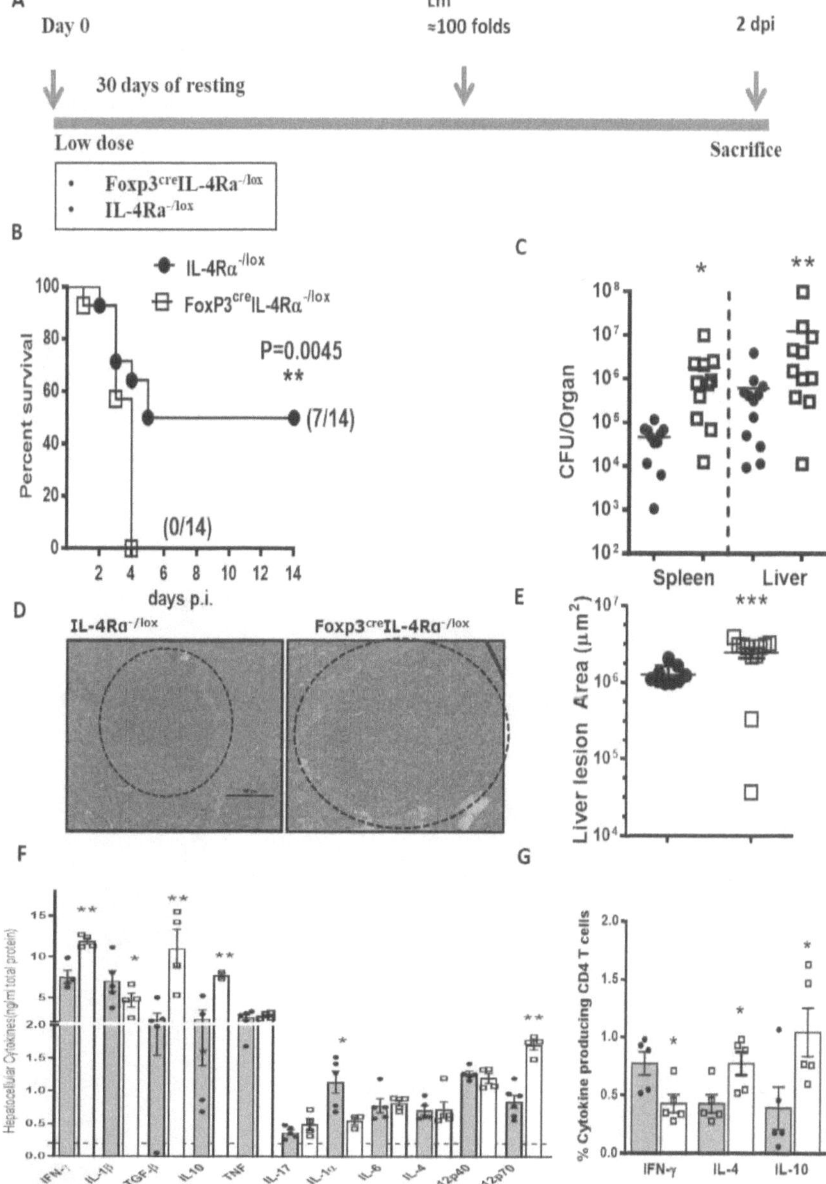

Figure 3.16 Increased Mortality and bacterial burden in Foxp3^{cre}IL-4Rα $^{-/lox}$ mice during *Lm* infection re-challenged: Mice were infected intraperitoneally with *Lm* with low dose *Lm* (1x10^4 CFU/mouse) and 30 days later re-challenged with 100-fold the initial dose (1x10^6). (A) Diagrammatic representation of secondary infection (B) Survival curves of mice, (C) spleen and liver *Lm* burden sacrificed 2 days post-challenge. (D) Formalin-fixed liver sections analysed for tissue pathology by H&E staining (circles indicating lesions). (E) Quantification of liver lesion size. (F) Liver homogenate cytokines of IFN-γ, IL-17, IL-1β, IL-1α, IL-6, TGF-β, IL-10, IL-4, TNF, IL-12p40, IL-12p70 (G) Splenic CD4$^+$ T cell producing cytokine of IFN-γ, IL-4, IL-10. Grey bars representing IL-4Rα$^{-/Lox}$ mice while white bars Foxp3^{cre}IL-4Rα$^{-/lox}$ mice Data represented as mean ± SEM of n= 5-6 mice/time point from two independent experiments and analysed by two-tailed, unpaired Student t-test (*p<0.05, **p<0.01, *** p < 0.001).

3.2.2 Introduction *Mtb* Section

In the previous section, we studied *Listeria monocytogenes (Lm)* as a model for the study of an intracellular pathogen. To further expand our knowledge on another intracellular pathogen of public health importance, we asked whether the IL-4Rα deletion on Foxp3 T reg cells could have similar effector function and phenotype during *Mtb* infection. *Mtb* is the causing agent of tuberculosis (TB). TB remains one of the greatest infectious diseases worldwide, with over 30% of individuals harbouring the microbe associated with huge mortality and morbidity (WHO 2018). The adaptive arm of immune sytem is essential for *Mtb* response during infection. During *Mtb* infection, T cell response is significantly delayed compared to other pathogens like *Lm*. This delay occurs at multiple stages including; late arrival of antigen-presenting dendritic cells carrying *Mtb* to the draining lymph nodes. The delayed proliferation of effector T-cells necessary for cytokine secretion. Also, this delay occurs due to the ability of *Mtb* to favour necrosis over apoptosis to escape from macrophage killing and delayed presentation to T cells (Larson *et al.* 2013). Foxp3 T reg has as function to suppress and dampens excessive immune responses but this role can be detrimental or beneficiary during infection depending on the disease model. T reg is recruited into the lungs during the first weeks of infection with less circulating T reg in the blood suggesting migration to the peripheral tissues (Burl *et al.* 2007). T reg migration to the peripheral tissues is a natural phenomenon in most diseases following infection and inflammation (Campbell & Koch 2011). A correlation between the T reg and the bacterial colony forming unit (CFU) has been established with excessive T reg playing a detrimental role in prohibiting action of pro-inflammatory cytokine effector killing (Marin *et al.* 2010). This has also been correlated by increased T reg at the site of caseating granuloma (Welsh *et al.* 2011). T reg effector balance is therefore tilted towards T effector function during *Mtb* infection, suggesting the infiltration of T reg may be detrimental during pulmonary TB (Welsh *et al.* 2011). T reg cells have the ability to suppress CD4$^+$ T cell function also, depletion of T reg cells during *in vitro* studies resulted in increased proliferation of T effector cells, that resulted in increased secretion of IFN-γ (Chen *et al.* 2007). Similarly, in mice studies depletion of T reg had a similar effect to *in vitro* studies (Fontenot *et al.* 2005; Kohm *et al.* 2006). To further validate the role of T reg in *Mtb* infection, sorted CD4$^+$CD25$^+$ (thymic T reg at naive state) and sorted CD4$^+$CD25$^-$ (effector T cells) have been shown to control *Mtb* differently. A significant decreased in bacterial burden in the effector population was witnessed compared to the (CD4$^+$CD25$^+$) T reg, suggesting a possible detrimental role of T reg during *Mtb* infections (Kursar *et al.* 2007). T reg plays a very important role in autoimmunity, targeting these population for complete deletion as an approach for host-directed therapy against *Mtb* is not tenable. Selective manipulation of this population without tempering with its principal function could be an alternative for host immunity control. To this effect, we targeted the IL-4Rα on Foxp3 cells to evaluate their gain/loss of function during *Mtb* infection in mouse.

Since our laboratory had previously shown that the absence of IL-4Rα on T reg during *Schistosoma mansoni* negatively influence the outcome of the disease (Aziz *et al.* 2018). This coupled with observed Th1 effector phenotype during *Lm* in mice could be a potential indicator or outcome in *Mtb* infection. Both TB and Listeriosis are intracellular pathogens and share similar immune responses up to certain extent however, pathogenesis is completely different.

Results

3.2.3 IL-4Rα transcript enhanced expression as a predictor during TB treatment

Whole transcriptomics via microarrays and RNA sequencing (RNA-Seq) techniques are regularly used to study gene expression profiling to holistically understand the host response to *Mtb* infection as a predictive tool to monitor TB disease, marker, treatment and/or outcome. Here, we exploited publicly available data on IL-4Rα and Foxp3 genes to understand the dynamics during the course of the disease in humans. The mRNA expression of the Il4rα gene in a South African cohort significantly increased in active TB patients (aTB) compared to latently infected TB controls (Figure 3.17A). Remarkably standard anti-TB treatment significantly reduced the expression of Il4rα in patients with TB after 48 weeks (Figure 3.17B), suggesting that IL-4Rα could be possibly used as a biomarker to evaluate the progression of treatment outcome. In addition to IL-4Rα, the expression of Foxp3 slightly increased during active TB (Figure 3.17C). During treatment; however, there were no significant differences during the course of treatment (Figure 3.17D). This suggests Foxp3 expression does not change during infection.

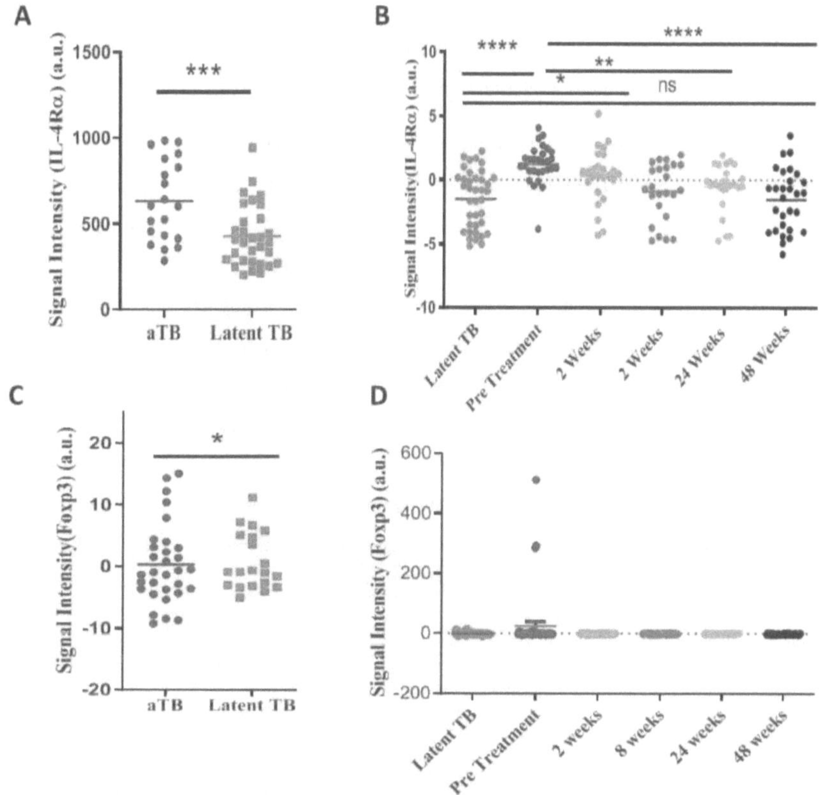

Figure 3.17: Transcriptional signature profile of Il4rα and Foxp3 mRNA in whole-blood of active TB and latently infected controls in the South African cohort. Il Il4rα and Foxp3 expression data from whole blood were sourced from publicly available dataset (A) gene expression of Il4rα, (C) Foxp3 in active TB and latently infected controls. Whole blood (B) Il4rα and (D) Foxp3 expression profile from a longitudinal cohort that follows up till the completion of anti-TB treatment. Data is generated by plotting signal intensity (a.u) and analysed by unpaired, Student t-test (A,C) and by one-way ANOVA with Turkey's multiple comparison test (B,D) (*p<0.05, **p<0.01, ***p<0.001, ****p<0.0001).

3.2.4 IL-4Rα signalling on Foxp3 is not decisive for *Mtb* bacterial burden and pathology control in mice

With a relatively stable expression of Foxp3 in the blood and differences in IL-4Rα expression during the course of treatment, we hypothesize that the deletion of IL-4Rα on Foxp3 T reg cells in mice affects the outcome of *Mtb* infection.

To elucidate the role of IL-4Rα signalling on Foxp3 T reg, mice were infected with a sub-lethal *Mtb* H37Rv at a dose of 100 CFU/mouse by aerosol. We performed survival studies and time course experiments to sacrifice at 3 and 18 weeks post-infection. We found no significant differences in bacterial burdens in the lungs and spleen at both 3 (Figure 3.18A) and 18 weeks (Figure 3.18B) post-infection. At these time points, lung histopathology was comparable between Foxp3^{cre}IL-4Rα$^{-/lox}$ mice measured by hematoxylin and eosin stain (H&E) (Figure 3.18E). Furthermore, quantification of free alveolar spaces to assess lung pathology and granuloma size did not reveal significant differences between groups (Figure 3.18F). To further investigate the effect on the survival of mice, we found no survival benefit (Figure 3.18C) and body weights change (Figure 3.18D) in these mice when compared to littermate control animals after 65 weeks. This suggests that deletion of IL-4Rα signalling on Foxp3 T regulatory cells have no effect during H37Rv infection.

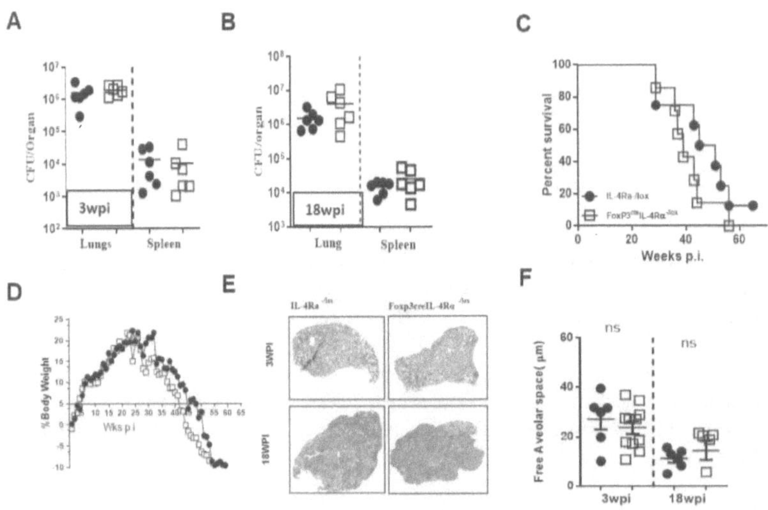

Figure 3.18 Deletion of IL-4Rα signalling on Foxp3^{cre}IL-4Rα$^{-/lox}$ mice does not alter bacterial burden and pathology: Control littermates (IL-4Rα$^{-/lox}$) and Foxp3^{cre} IL-4Rα$^{-/lox}$ mice were infected by

aerosol with 100 CFU/mouse of *Mtb* H37Rv (n=6 mice/group) mice sacrificed at 3 and 18 weeks post-infection (wpi). (A) The bacterial burden of lungs and spleen at 3 wpi, (B) bacterial burden at 18 wpi, (C) survival curve for 65 weeks post-infection. (D) Body-weight change for the mortality study. (E) Representative image of H&E histopathology staining, (F) quantification of alveolar spaces. Error bars signify mean ± SEM. Data revealed are representative of two independent experiments. Data is analysed using unpaired, student t-test*, P≤0.05; **, P ≤ 0.01; ***, P≤0.001.

3.2.5 Foxp3^{cre}IL-4Rα$^{-/lox}$ mice had no effect in lung cytokine profile relative to littermate control during *Mtb* infection

We investigated whether the absence of IL-4Rα on Foxp3 T reg mice (Foxp3^{cre}IL-4Rα$^{-/lox}$) on the lung cytokine profile in tissue homogenates, at 3 and 18wpi. We found a significant decrease in Nitric oxide (NO) in the Foxp3^{cre}IL-4Rα$^{-/lox}$ mice, this may explain an increasing trend in bacterial burdens. However, there was a slight increase in IGF-1 and IL-23 at 18wpi in the Foxp3^{cre}IL-4Rα$^{-/lox}$ mice at both time points. The role of IGF-1 in *Mtb* infection has not been well documented. IL-23 has been shown to contribute to initiation Th17 responses however, IL-17 was not affected. The role of IL-17 during *Mtb* infection is not well understood. During BCG vaccination, no differences in IL-17 have been observed (Gopal *et al.* 2012) however IL-17 in chronic stages of TB can contribute to pathological inflammation (Cruz *et al.* 2010). There was an impaired production of GM-CSF in the Foxp3^{cre}IL-4Rα$^{-/lox}$ mice, GM-CSF signalling is known to be highly activated during *Mtb* infection. However, neutralising GM-CSF had no effect on bacterial burden in mice models. Lack of GM-CSF led to increasing in granuloma formations in mice models (Benmerzoug *et al.* 2018) but increased GM-CSF concentrations had no major effect. Furthermore, no differences were observed in IL-12p40, IL-17, IL-4, IFN-γ, IL-12p70, IL-6, IL-1α, IL-10 and TGF-β at both time points (3 and 18wpi). Furthermore, we examined the chemokines CXCL1, CCL3, CXCL10, CXCL2 and found no differences. However, there was an increase in CXCL5 at 3wpi for the Foxp3^{cre}IL-4Rα$^{-/lox}$ mice. Overall, this shows that absence of IL-4Rα signalling on Foxp3 T regulatory cells did not have significant differences in cytokines.

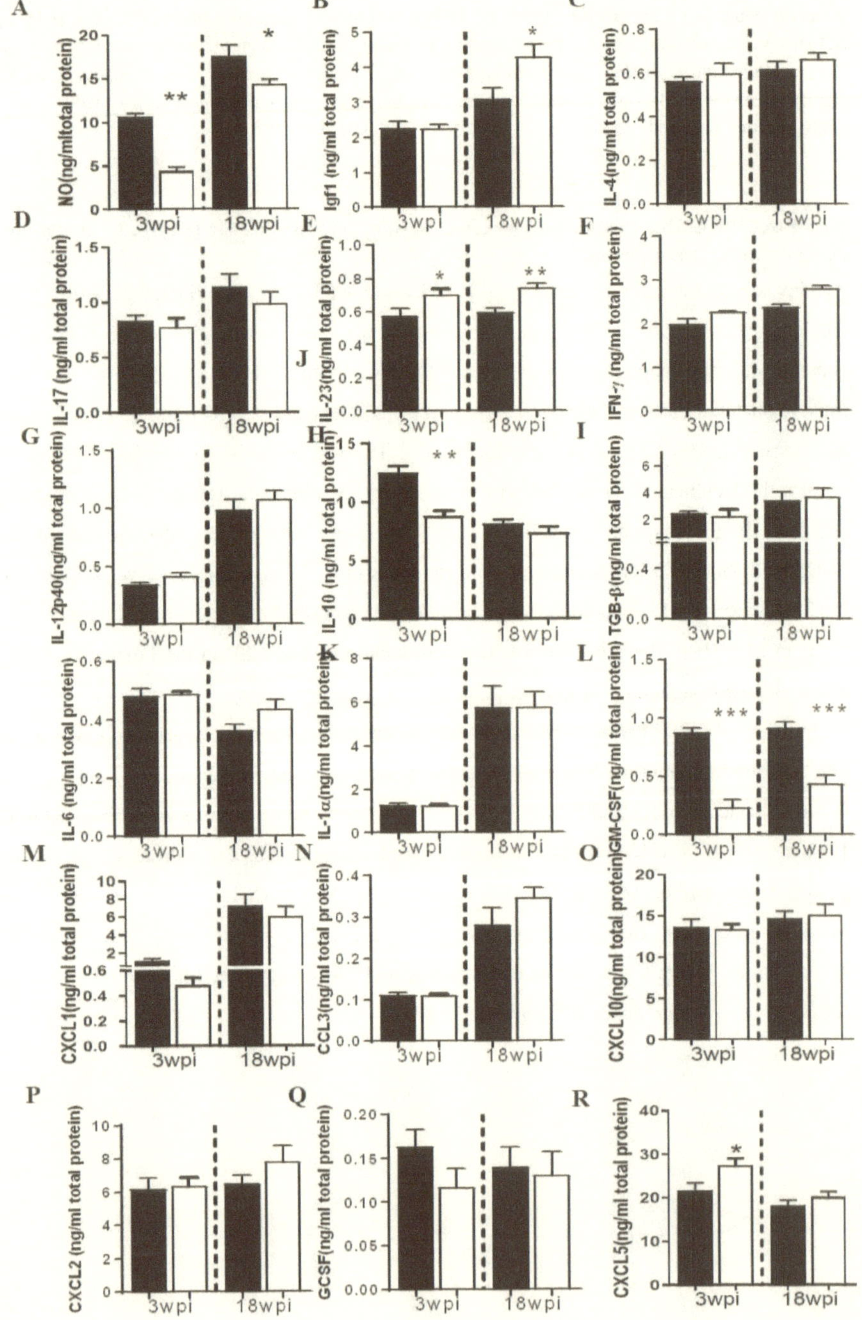

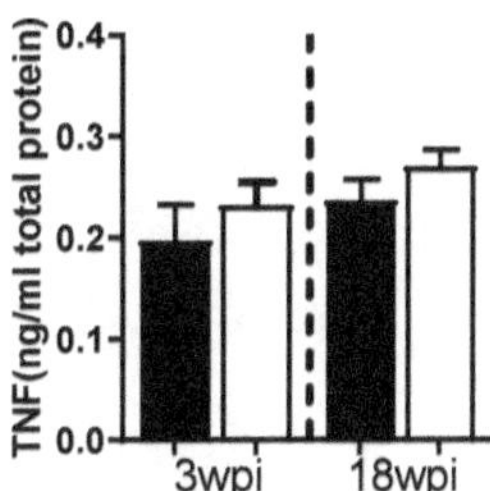

Figure 3.19: Lung homogenate cytokine/chemokine profiles in *Mtb* H37Rv infected Foxp3creIL-4Rα -/lox mice and littermate control. Mice were infected with 100 CFU/mouse with *Mtb* H37Rv by aerosol and sacrificed at 3wpi and 18wpi, and lung cytokines were determined by ELISA: (A) Nitrite Oxide(NO), (B) Igf1, (C) IL-4, (D) IL-17, (E) IL-23, (F) IFN-γ, (G) IL-12p40, (H) IL-10, (I) TGF-β, (J) IL-6,(K) IL-1α, (L) GM-CSF, (M) CXCL1, (N) CCL3, (O) CXCL10, (P) CXCL2,(Q) GCSF (R) CXCL5. (S) and TNF Error bars signify mean ± SEM. These results are an illustration of two similar experiments. Data is analysed using unpaired, student t-test *, P≤0.05; **, P ≤ 0.01; ***, P≤0.001;

3.2.6 Cytokine production from mediastinal lymph nodes shows a pro-inflammatory cytokine profile in Foxp3creIL-4Rα -/lox mice.

Mediastinal lymph nodes are the most commonly infected organ apart from the lungs during *Mtb* infection. Cross-talking between the antigen-presenting cells and T cells and consequent activation is initiated at the mediastinal lymph nodes. We collected lymph nodes from *Mtb*-H37Rv infected mouse at 3 and 18wpi, surface stained for CD4+ T cells and CD8+ T cells. Intracellular cytokine staining was performed after *ex vivo* stimulation. Though no major differences were observed for the immune cell frequencies at the lungs, we pursue the lymph node where deletion IL-4Rα on T regs was pronounced. No significant differences in CD4+ T cell cytokines were observed at 3wpi with IFN-γ, IL-10, and IL-4. At 18 wpi, CD4+ T and CD8+ T cells were analysed for IFN-γ, IL-2, IL-17, TNF, IL-4, and IL-10 production. Cells were stimulated with *Mtb* cell lysate (H37Rv, BEI Resources) or PMA/Ionomycin followed by Monensin blockade or left unstimulated. Foxp3creIL-4Rα-/lox mice showed no differences in IFN-γ, IL-2, IL-17, TNF, IL-4 and IL-10 cytokine secretion when left unstimulated on both CD4 + T cells (Figure 3.20A) and CD8+ T cells (Figure 3.20D). However, as expected with H37Rv lysate stimulation, CD4+ T cells produced significantly higher IFN-γ, IL-17 and TNF in Foxp3creIL-4Rα-/lox mice (Figure 3.20 B) and CD8+ T cells decreased IL-4 and IL-10 (Figure

3.20E). Stimulation with PMA/ionomycin led to significant secretion of IL-17 and TNF for CD4$^+$ T cells (Figure 3.20C) and a significant increase in IFN-γ and TNF levels for CD8 T cells (Figure 3.20F). Similarly to Listeriosis, the deletion of the IL-4Rα on Foxp3 T cells was more significant in the lymph nodes suggesting more activity at the secondary lymphoid organs. This increased IFN-γ, IL-17 and TNF cytokines secretion by Foxp3^{cre}IL-4Rα$^{-/lox}$ T lymphocytes suggest an effector function as a result of IL-4Rα deletion on T reg.

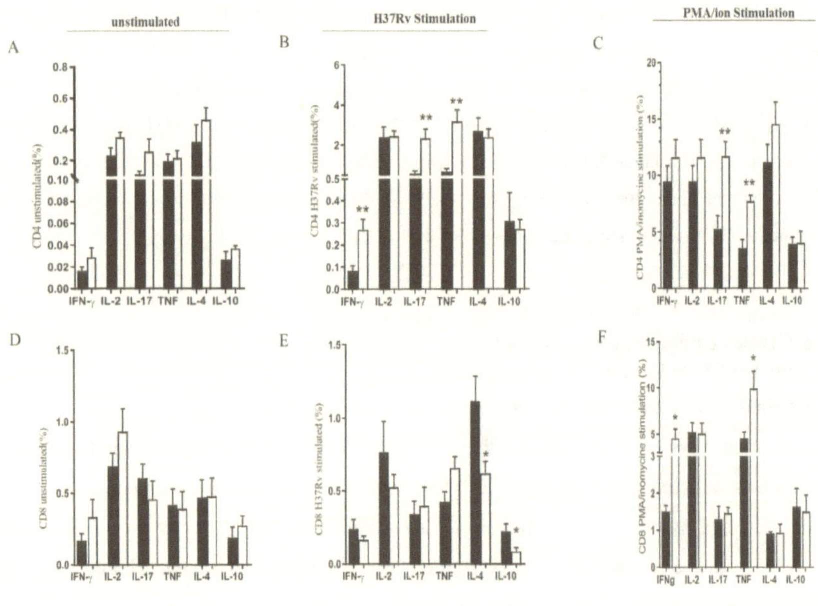

Figure 3.20: Intracellular cytokine profile in mediastinal lymph node T cells during *Mtb* infection: Mice were infected by aerosol and sacrificed at 18wpi. A single-cell suspension of total mediastinal lymph nodes was prepared, and 2 million cells were then seeded to either to determine the frequency of cytokine production IFN-γ, IL-2, Il-17, TNF, IL-4 and IL-10 (A&D) cells in media, (B&E) after H37Rv lysate stimulation, and (G&F) after PMA/ionomycin stimulation. Results represent 6 mice per group and representative of two experiments. White bars represent Foxp3^{cre}IL-4Rα$^{-/lox}$ while black bars their littermate control (IL-4Rα$^{-/Lox}$). Data are denoted as mean ± SEM, analysed using unpaired, student t-test, * p < 0.05, ** p < 0.01, ***p <0.001.

3.2.7 Deletion of IL-4Rα on Foxp3 T reg cells influences immune cellular population lymph node in early H37Rv *Mtb* infections.

To further understand whether the abrogation of IL-4Rα signalling on Foxp3 T reg alters the immune cell populations at 3 wpi. Mediastinal lymph nodes were harvested and stained for the presence of myeloid and lymphoid cells and acquired on the Fortessa. There was a significant increase in total cell numbers in Foxp3^{cre}IL-4Rα$^{-/lox}$ mice (Figure 3.21A) suggesting increased infiltration of immune cells into the lymph nodes early during infection at 3wpi. No differences were observed in the myeloid populations (Figure 3.21B). A significant increase in CD4$^+$ and CD8$^+$ T cells at the mediastinum lymph node (Figure 3.21C). We next sought to investigate if the deletion of IL-4Rα on T reg affected naïve; effector and central memory CD4 T cells in the Foxp3^{cre}IL-4Rα $^{-/lox}$ mice. There was a significant increase in CD4 effector T cells in the Foxp3^{cre}Il-4Rα$^{-/lox}$. These results suggest the absence of IL-4Rα signalling on Foxp3 T regulatory T cells increased CD4 and CD8 T cell recruitment in early *Mtb* infection.

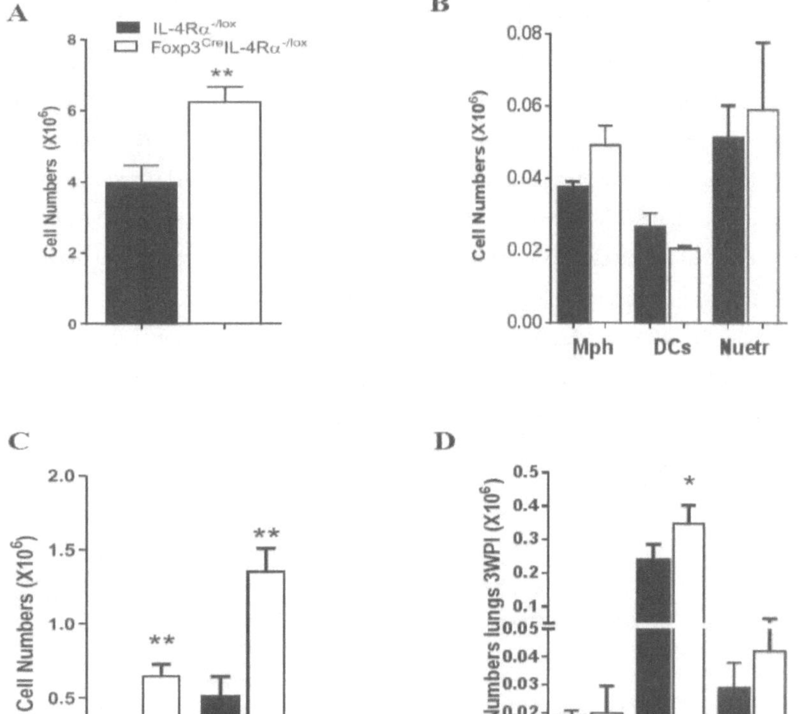

Figure 3.21: Cellular population of lymph node in Foxp3creIl-4Rα-/lox mice during *Mtb* infection at 3 wpi: Mice were infected with low dose (100CFU/mouse) H37Rv and sacrificed at 3wpi to determine immune cell using flow cytometry and analysed with Flowjo to quantify the populations in mediastinal lymph node. (A) Mediastinal lymph node total cell numbers (B) myeloid cell population (C) CD8/CD4 T cell population (D) mediastinal lymph node naïve, central, and effector T cell subsets. Results are representative of two independent experiments (n=5-6 per group) Error bars signify mean ± SEM. Data revealed are representative of two independent experiments. Data is analysed using unpaired, student t-test;*, P≤0.05; **, P ≤ 0.01; ***, P≤0.001;

3.2.8 I IL-4Rα-mediated signalling on Foxp3 T reg cells influences the immune cell population in lymph node in chronic *Mtb* infection.

Similar to the acute stage (3wpi), we sought to determine the immune cell populations at a chronic stage (18wpi) of Mtb infection. Mediastinal lymph node single-cell suspension was obtained and stained for myeloid and lymphoid cell populations. No differences in the cell numbers in the lymph node were observed (Figure 3.22A). Similar to 3wpi, there were no differences in the myeloid population (Macrophages, dendritic cells, and neutrophils) (Figure 3.22B), however consistent with 3wpi, a significant increase in CD8$^+$ and CD4$^+$ T cell population in the lymph node for the Foxp3^{cre}Il-4R$\alpha^{-/lox}$ mice (Figure 3.22C). We observed a significant increase in the effector and central CD4$^+$ T cell memory in FoxP3^{cre}IL-4R$\alpha^{-/lox}$ mice compared to littermate control (Figure 3.22D, E and F). The increase in effector CD4 T cells correlated with an increase in different intracellular cytokines observed during this time. These results suggest that the absence of IL-4Rα signalling on T reg possibly affects effector T cells at the mediastinal lymph nodes that translate into augmented cytokine production.

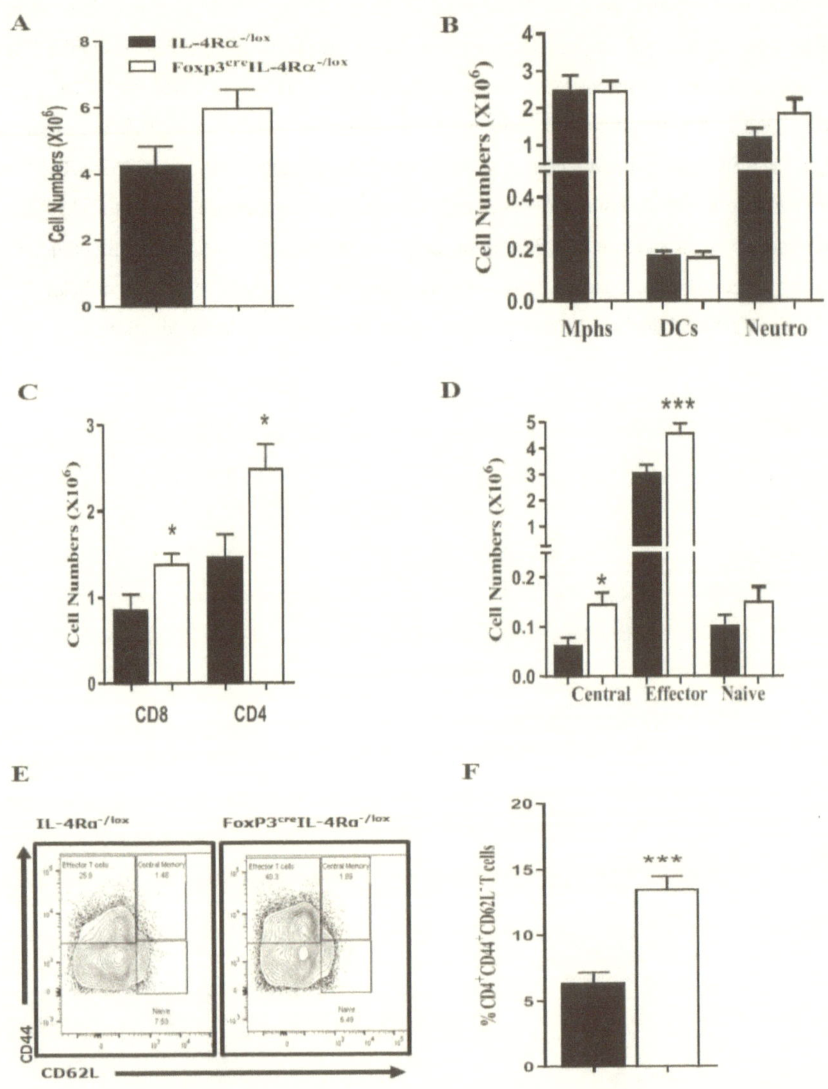

Figure 3.22 Cellular population of Foxp3^{cre}Il-4Rα^{-/lox} mice during *Mtb* infection at 18 wpi: Mice were infected with low dose (100CFU/mouse) H37Rv and sacrificed at 18 wpi to determine immune cell using Flow cytometry and analysed with Flowjo population in mediastinal lymph node. (A) Total

cell numbers (B) myeloid population (C) CD8/CD4 T cell population (D) CD4 T effector, naïve and central cell numbers (E) Represented percentage of flow cytometry of CD4 T effector naïve, Central cells (F) Mediastinal lymph cell numbers Naïve, Central, Effector T cell. Results are representative of two independent experiments (n=5-6 per group) Error bars signify mean ± SEM. Data is analysed using unpaired, student t-test.*, P≤0.05; **, P ≤ 0.01; ***, P≤0.001.

CHAPTER 4:
DISCUSSION

The *Listeria monocytogenes* infection in mice model has been widely studied to understand the immunological responses against intracellular pathogens (Pamer 2004; Hamon *et al.* 2006). To understand the basic mechanisms of immune responses to pathogenesis, we use *Lm* and *Mtb* infections in mice model for possible translation into therapeutic and vaccine approaches. These models are commonly used to assess the Th1 immune responses to inflammation. These two models are related and *Lm* is used to understand T cell dynamics. Recent studies have shown the use of *Lm* strains fused with ESAT-6 protein of *Mtb* for the design of safety and a protective vaccine against tuberculosis (Yin *et al.* 2017).

During *Lm* infection in mice, early control is carried out by the innate immunity most notable the neutrophils and macrophages which account for bacterial killing (Seki *et al.* 2002; Witter *et al.* 2016; Lücke *et al.* 2018). However, despite this important role by myeloid cells, a potent T cell response is necessary for maintained clearance and development of life-long protective immunity, largely orchestrated by CD8$^+$ T cells (Busch *et al.* 1998; Sun & Bevan 2003). CD8$^+$ T cells recognise *Lm* in the cytosol and induce clearance, while the CD4$^+$ T cell response maintains a robust memory T cell responses and confer sterilizing immunity (Harty & Badovinac 2002; Lara-Tejero & Pamer 2004). CD4$^+$ T cells produce Th1 cytokines mainly IL-12, IFN-γ and TNF that mediate the potentiation of *Lm* clearance (Hsieh *et al.* 1993). T cells specific response analysis involves a more complex differentiation and contraction of T cells into effector and central memory which are important for clearance after reinfection (Mercado *et al.* 2000). T cells plasticity allows them to change to various T cell subsets in response to pathogens with cytokine production. This event is flexible, extraordinarily diverse, and not terminally differentiated as previously thought (Talwar *et al.* 2013). This trend of events is defined by transcriptional factors such as signal transducer activator of transcription (STAT-1) and T box (t-bet) which are biased towards a Th1 response. Similarly, STAT-6 and STAT-5, control the master Th2 GATA-3 transcriptional factor (Annunziato & Romagnani 2009). Th1/Th2 lineages are associated with the production of IFN-γ and IL-4 cytokines respectively (Arun *et al.* 2011). Th17 cells are characterised by the retinoic acid-related orphan receptor (RORγt) transcriptional factor signature and produce IL-17, plasticity from Th17 to T reg with Forkhead box P3 (Foxp3) have been shown to alter among them depending on the conditions (Sawant & Vignali 2014). TGF-β, IL-4, and IL-23 have been shown to drive Th17 to T reg cells while IL-5 and IL-21 have been shown to move from T reg to Th17 cells (Lee *et al.*

2009). Th17 cells enhanced Th1 cells mediated by IL-12 cytokine environment (Lee *et al.* 2009; Bending *et al.* 2009). Foxp3 regulatory T cells have been shown to undergo plasticity to a Th1 or Th2 depending on the cytokine milieu (Komatsu *et al.* 2009; Zhou *et al.* 2009). Studies have clearly shown a detrimental role of T reg cells during certain bacterial infection, due to simultaneous expansion of Th1 and T reg. (Scott-Browne *et al.* 2007; Shafiani *et al.* 2010; Johanns *et al.* 2010; Rowe *et al.* 2011)

Recently, the role of IL-4Rα on Foxp3 T regulatory cells was established on Th2 disease models. IL-4Rα on T reg was required for the conversion of T reg cells to Th2 cells in vitro and *in vivo* during *Heligmosomoides polygyrus* infection (Pelly *et al.* 2017). Furthermore, during *Schistosoma mansoni* infection, IL-4Rα signalling on Foxp3 T reg cells was demonstrated to be necessary to control exacerbated inflammation (Aziz *et al.* 2018). However, the role of IL-4Rα on Foxp3 T reg cells on *Lm* and *Mtb* infection has not been elucidated. In this study, we asked whether deletion of IL-4Rα on Foxp3 T cells effects the effector/Treg balance during *Lm* and *Mtb* infections. The proportion of T reg and effector T cells can define the outcome of infection.

The Lack of human cohort studies on Listeriosis due to the inability to trace the source of infection and the difficulty of estimating incubation periods (Goulet *et al.* 2013) warranted us to use transcriptional mice studies to understand the dynamics of the expression of mRNA IL-4Rα/Foxp3 in spleen and liver, over the course of infection. (Figure 3.1). Significant increase in IL-4Rα expression during the disease progression shows the dynamics during infection. We, therefore, choose acute (3 days) and chronic (7 days) post-infection reflective of innate and adaptive phases of the disease for *Lm in vivo* infections (Busch *et al.* 1998; Zenewicz & Shen 2007). These dynamics were similar to *Mtb*-infected human cohort studies which showed increased expression of IL-4Rα mRNA in blood of TB (Berry *et al.* 2010; Maertzdorf *et al.* 2011; Bloom *et al.* 2013; Cliff *et al.* 2013).

The role of IL-4 and IL-13 as type 2 cytokines which are pivotal in antagonising Th1 cytokines. However, the role of IL-4 on T regs remains inconclusive. Studies have suggested beneficial role of IL-4 on CD4$^+$ CD25$^+$ T regs (Prochazkova *et al.* 2009).On the other hand IL-4 presence depends the differentiation process of induced Tregs thereby deregulating their Foxp3 function (Dardalhon *et al.* 2008). The absence of IL-4Rα on Foxp3 T reg cells during *in vivo* settings led to a better understanding of the necessity of these cells during the clearance or reduction in bacterial burdens, and also on the survival of the mice during *Lm* infection. Interestingly, this result tie with studies in which IL-4 production was considered harmful during listeriosis in mice (Emoto *et al.* 1997). IL-4 signalling has been considered detrimental during *Lm* infection since prior administration of anti-IL-4 antibody to mice drives bacterial clearance during *Lm* infection in mice (Haak-Frendscho *et al.* 1992; Wagner & Czuprynski 1993; Szalay *et al.* 1996). This dynamics of IL-4/IL-4Rα on *Lm* has been demonstrated only on a global knockout or transient ablation using anti-IL-4. Our laboratory has recently focused more on exploring and unravelling a novel role of cell-specific IL-4Rα knockdown in different disease models such as schistosomiasis (Aziz *et al.* 2018), allergy (in preparation) as well as *Lm* and *Mtb* infections which are the main focus of this project.

In order to better understand this phenomenon, we observed the quality of Foxp3 was significantly decreased in mouse lacking IL-4Rα on Foxp3 T regulatory cells, signifying that IL-4Rα is required to maintain the stability and probably the function of T regulatory cells during *Lm* infection. The quality of Foxp3 T cells is affected by signals from antigen, and cytokines production (Dowling *et al.* 2018). The decrease of Foxp3 T cells tilts and strengthens the immune balance to an effector Th1 phenotype which is fundamental for *Lm* pathogenic clearance (Zenewicz & Shen 2007). This was quite remarkable when we found a significant decrease in the expression of Foxp3 at 3 dpi (Figure 3.3A) and 7 dpi (Figure 3.3B) in the spleen, but not in the liver tissue. This suggests that although the Foxp3 T regulatory population is not affected by the loss of IL-4Rα at a steady-state, during infection the quality and possibly the function of Foxp3 T regs are affected. Foxp3 instability has shown transient changes from Foxp3 T cells to Th2 (exFoxp3 T cells), which proliferates in tissues and produce inflammatory cytokines (Zhou *et al.* 2009). Furthermore, we observed a significant increase in T-bet in the Foxp3^{cre}Il-4Rα$^{-/lox}$ mice, demonstrating a possible indicator of enhanced Th1 due to loss of Foxp3 T cell population. This is speculative since we did not use a multigene reporter and fate-reporter sysytems mice to demonstrate the shift from Foxp3 regulatory T cells to exFoxp3 (Th1) as in *Heligmosomoides polygyrus* infection which to show a shift from exFoxp3 to Th2 (Pelly *et al.* 2017). Tilting this balance has been shown to play an important beneficiary function most notable in *Listeria monocytogenes*, and *Salmonella enterica* where near-total depletion of Foxp3 T reg cells was achieved (Johanns *et al.* 2010; Rowe *et al.* 2011, 2012). However, we demonstrated that the lack of stability was due to the loss of IL-4Rα, the effector T cells in Foxp3^{cre}IL-4Rα$^{-/lox}$ mice were significantly increased during *Lm* infections, therefore, asserting the imbalance witnessed. This interplay is fundamental as the ratio of regulatory CD4[+] T cells and the effector immune cells are key to host response (Wing & Sakaguchi 2010). Foxp3 regulatory T cells population is also known to impede the priming of effector T cells (Ertelt *et al.* 2009, 2011; Eisenstein & Williams 2009; Omenetti & Pizarro 2015).

IL-4Rα signalling on T reg cells is essential to maintain T reg and loss of IL-4Rα on T reg leads to increase CD8[+]T cells in Foxp3[cre]IL-4Rα[-/lox] mice. IL-12 IFN-β, IFN-α, secreted from myeloid cells, which are able to activate CD8[+] T cells and expansion *in vitro,* however, in *in vivo* setting, these cytokines where non-essential towards the activation and expansion of CD8[+] T cells in *Lm* infection *in vivo,* (Curtsinger *et al.* 2003, 2005). Previously, it has been reported that during *Lm* infection Foxp3 T reg cells' impeded the activation and expansion of CD8[+]T cells, and deletion of T reg leads to expansion of CD8[+] T cells (Ertelt *et al.* 2011). We observed a significant increase in CD8[+] T cells when IL-4Rα was absent on Foxp3 T cells. CD8[+] T cells are very crucial for *Lm* infection (Tvinnereim *et al.* 2002; Shedlock *et al.* 2003; Hamon *et al.* 2006; Zaiss *et al.* 2008; Condotta *et al.* 2012) This possibly explain the reduced listerial burdens, we observed in Foxp3[cre]IL-4Rα[-/lox] mice.

CD8[+] T cells are known to secrete granzyme B and perforin during effector function and vaccination of host, which is developed during CD8[+] T cell proliferation into cytolytic T lymphocytes in response to antigen (Mouchacca *et al.* 2013). This is achieved by the directed release of granzyme B by CD8[+] T cells, though mechanistically, the deficiency of IFN-γ as an effector cytokine affects killing during primary infection more than the immediate of the direct effect of granzyme B (Messingham *et al.* 2007). So, though we experienced higher secretion of granzyme B, we rather looked for the expression of IFN-γ in splenic T cells during this time frame. At 7 dpi *Lm* infection, there was a significant increase in IFN-γ in the serum, increase in IFN-γ upon αCD3 re-stimulation of the splenocytes and IFN-γ produced by CD4[+] and CD8[+]T cells. Increased splenic IFN-γ at day 6 post-infection has been shown to correlate with clearance of *Lm* in the spleen and peritoneal cavity, though IFN-γ secretion was not exclusively secreted by T cells, with the early release coming from NK cells (Buchmeier & Schreiber 1985; van Dissel *et al.* 1987; Thäle & Kiderlen 2005). Similar to granzyme B, IFN-γ, secretion alone is necessary but not indispensable for host killing effect. (Leenen *et al.* 1994). At 3dpi, we did not observe significant differences in the levels of in IFN-γ, IL-10, and TNF. At 7dpi, there was a significant increase in IFN-γ and IL-10 when stimulated with anti-CD3 and a similar trend was observed in HKLM stimulation at 7 dpi (Figure 3.7D-E). This might explain a modest effect in bacterial burdens and histology on day 3, and hence the cytokines. However, the major cytokine differences were observed at day 7 was IL-2 which was significantly increased concomitantly with IFN-γ upon stimulations. IL-2 controls the expression of transcriptional factors, hence contributing to Th1 cell development (Liao *et al.* 2011). It is also known to maintain T reg cells and effector T cell differentiation and control of cytokine secretion (Wang & Secombes 2013; Arenas-Ramirez *et al.* 2015; Mitra & Leonard 2018). IL-2 significantly increased in the Foxp3^{cre} IL-4Rα$^{-/lox}$ mice during *Lm* infection was also correlated with effector and Th1 cytokines as described above with conspicuous T-bet Th1 transcriptional factor. IL-2 is known to maintain the functional stability of T reg, though there were decreased in T reg during infection, the increase in IL-2 probably helped maintain T reg cells that had lost the IL-4R.

The innate response was affected by the absence of IL-4Rα on Foxp3. Primary infection is fought by the myeloid cells in the spleen and liver by the splenic marginal zone of the red pulp (Conlan 1997; Condotta *et al.* 2012), but the T-zone of the white pulp is where effector T cells probably cross-talk with dendritic cells (Aoshi *et al.* 2008; Edelson *et al.* 2011). In Foxp3^{cre}IL-4Rα$^{-/lox}$ mice, we observed less destruction of white pulp during *Lm* infection suggesting improved control during an adaptive response. Cellular depletion of white pulp during *Lm* infection indicated a critical role of myelomonocytic cells interactions with CD8 T cells at effector (Waite *et al.* 2011). An increase in neutrophils at both time points was also observed in Foxp3^{cre}Il-4Rα$^{-/lox}$ mice. Neutrophils are known to play an important protective role by producing cytokines that potentiate killing of the *Lm* (Carr *et al.* 2011; Witter *et al.* 2016). Neutrophils are known to appear within the first 24 hours and depletion using monoclonal antibodies concluded that the neutrophils are essential during *Lm* infection. (Rogers & Unanue 1993; Conlan & North 1994; Czuprynski *et al.* 1994; Conlan 1997). The use of anti-Ly6G monoclonal antibody for neutrophils has also established this role of neutrophils (Edelson *et al.* 2011a; Carr *et al.* 2011). Increase in neutrophils, in Foxp3^{cre}IL-4Rα$^{-/lox}$ mice increase could possibly explain reduced bacterial burden as well as cellular infiltration in histopathology of spleen and liver. This suggests that there was increased recruitment of immune cells in the spleen, this was also true for inflammatory macrophages (7dpi) in the Foxp3^{cre}IL-4Rα$^{-/lox}$ (Figure 3.9) in which we observed and significant increase. At the liver, there was less recruitment of macrophages at both time points. IL-12 secreted by macrophages and NK cells promote the development of Th1 cells, whereas IL-4 is well known for the development of Th2 cells. (Bancroft *et al.* 1991; Hsieh *et al.* 1993; Scott 1993; Locksley 1993; Seder & Paul 1994*b*). There was a slight increase in the recruitment dendritic cells at the early time point (3dpi) for the Foxp3^{cre}IL-4Rα$^{-/lox}$ mice in the spleen, however, no differences were observed in both groups at the later time point. Neutrophils (GR1^{+}CD11b^{+}Cd11C^{-}) were also significantly increased at the spleen but not in liver for the Foxp3^{cre}IL-4Rα$^{-/lox}$ mice. The role of neutrophils in diseases has been shown to be both detrimental and protective depending on the disease.

During vaccination and re-challenged (Figure 3.15), infection with of Foxp3^{cre}Il-4Rα$^{-/lox}$ mice with *Lm* revealed a totally different phenotype on the role of IL-4Rα on Foxp3. The Foxp3^{cre}IL-4Rα$^{-/lox}$ mice were highly susceptible compared to primary infection. (Figure 3.4). A possible explanation is that *Lm* infection is a fast model (adaptive immunity sets in 4 to 5days) (Zenewicz & Shen 2007). During the primary phase, the absence of the receptor affects the dynamics of Foxp3 T cells (Figure 3.3). This affects the expression of cytokines, most notable IFN-γ at the spleen (Figures 3.7, 3.8 and 3.10). Secretion of IFN-γ has a beneficiary effect during *Lm* infection (Haak-Frendscho *et al.* 1992; Szalay *et al.* 1996; Andersson *et al.* 1998; Thäle & Kiderlen 2005; Messingham *et al.* 2007; Yin *et al.* 2017). However, protracted infection, the loss of IL-4Rα and the resultant effect on the Foxp3 become detrimental as evidenced on longer models (Pelly *et al.* 2017; Aziz *et al.* 2018). This susceptibility was matched with increased spleen and liver burdens and H&E histopathology. A significant amount of IFN-γ, IL-10, TGF-β and IL-12p40 was secreted in liver homogenate cytokine of Foxp3^{cre}Il-4Rα$^{-/lox}$ mice. The observation consistent with Aziz and colleagues, where they described a significant increase of cytokines in the liver, possibly accounting for tissue damage. In addition, at the spleen, there was a reduced secretion of IFN-γ with a corresponding increased secretion of immunosuppressive cytokines, a possible indication of inhibition of IFN-γ. In the absence of CD4^{+} T cells, naïve CD8^{+} T cells respond very well to *Lm* infection during primary infection and clear off *Lm*, however, during secondary immunization mice lacking CD4^{+} T cells with potent CD8^{+} T cell memory showed defective ability to respond to a second encounter with the antigen (Sun & Bevan 2003). Due to loss of IL-4Rα on CD4^{+} T Foxp3 regulatory T cells, this may have affected CD4 T cells hence during rechallenge could not mount a sustainable control similar primary infection.

In order to mechanistically determine the phenotype observed during primary *Lm*, co-culture of T cells derived from Foxp3^{cre}Il-4Rα$^{-/lox}$ mice with Listeria (HKLM) exposed macrophages

(BMDM) were cultured in the presence of HKLM antigen for during 72 hours. T regs (CD4$^+$CD25$^+$) cells from sorted for Foxp3^{cre}Il-4Rα$^{-/lox}$ mice showed significant CD4 T cell effector (CD44$^+$CD62L$^-$) phenotype, similar to *in vivo* listeriosis and tuberculosis. Interesting the percentage of CD4$^+$Foxp3$^+$ T cells was also significantly reduced from cells from sorted from Foxp3^{cre}Il-4Rα$^{-/lox}$ mice in conformity with Foxp3 cells in Figure 3. This translate into a loss of IL-4Rα on Foxp3 T cells results in reduced Foxp3 expression in Foxp3^{cre}Il-4Rα$^{-/lox}$ mice and more effector function. This is reflective in studies where CD4$^+$CD25$^+$ has been shown to suppress Foxp3 expression during *Lm* infection (Hussain & Paterson 2004; Ma *et al.* 2007; Ertelt *et al.* 2009a). Quite interestingly, the amount of IL-10 was significantly decreased in Foxp3^{cre}IL-4Rα$^{-/lox}$ mice (Figure 15I). Suggesting less suppressive activity of IL-10 during *Lm* infection.(Laidlaw *et al.* 2015). This was quite expected as we had more effector T cells in Foxp3^{cre}Il-4Rα$^{-/lox}$ mice. However, we did not observe any difference in IFN-γ (Figure 3.15H) *in vivo*, suggesting other factors and/or source of cytokine play a role in to IFN-γ secretion.

During *Mtb* infection with H37Rv, we did not observe any differences in bacterial loads during the acute and chronic phase of infection (Figure 3.17). However, deletion of IL-4/IL-4Rα in mice studies have demonstrated varying results. For example, during *L. major* IR17 3 infection, IL-4$^{-/-}$ deletion in mice demonstrated control of the parasite through IL-4Rα, this was not through an alternative shift in Th1 with the production of IFN-γ during the acute infection (Noben-Trauth *et al.* 1999) However, IL-4 secretion during the chronic stage suppressed host protective Th1 response (Biedermann *et al.* 2001). Increase of IL-4 cytokine production from CD4$^+$ and CD8$^+$ T cells have increased with patients with pulmonary tuberculosis (van Crevel *et al.* 2000; Ordway *et al.* 2005; Mihret *et al.* 2012). In *Mtb* infection IL-4$^{-/-}$ mice or IL-4 neutralisation using antibodies has been shown to result in reduced bacterial loads and improved histopathology (Hernandez-Pando *et al.* 2004; Roy *et al.* 2008). Additionally, the use of neutralising anti-IL-4 antibody administered in mice during early or late stages have been shown significant reduction in bacterial burden (Roy *et al.* 2008), suggesting the shift in the Th1/Th2 axis may play a potential role in effector killing during infection. Our results did not confirm to this paradigm. A possible explanation is likely different pathogenesis, slowly growing nature of *Mtb* in addition to likely the less virulence of the H37Rv strain. In BALB/c mice, and in humans studies, *Mtb* infection is associated with increase in the levels of IL-4 from CD4$^+$ T cells and CD8$^+$ T cells during the chronic phases (Seah *et al.* 2000; van Crevel *et al.* 2000; Smith *et al.* 2002; Lienhardt *et al.* 2002). Consistently, in human cohort studies, we found increased IL-4Rα mRNA transcripts from the publicly available datasets. In human cohort studies, there was a significant increase in the IL-4α receptor in active TB patients compared to latent patients. This was similar to the Gambia cohorts and the UK cohort. Though the increase in all cohorts, was significant, increases in African cohorts have been suggested to emanate from concomitant helminths infections in these settings more than in the UK settings (Rook *et al.* 2004). Pre-existing helminths have been shown to inhibit pulmonary anti-TB defence by the IL-4Rα signalling (Potian *et al.* 2011). IL-4Rα decreased during the course of treatment and reverted to the levels of latently infected control individuals prior to treatment, suggesting the Il-4Rα could be used as a potential marker to monitor the progression to disease.

Loss of IL-4Rα on Foxp3 T regulatory cells diminished the quality measured with geometric fluorescent intensity (GMFI) of Foxp3. Most interestingly, this also translated into an effector T cell balance during *Mtb* infection. This confirmed the fact that decrease in Foxp3 T cells shifts the balance, confirming the role of IL-4Rα on the stability of T regulatory cell population. To better confirmed this, mediastinum lymph node stimulation with H37Rv lysate and PMA/ionomycin. This led to a significant increase in CD4+ T cell producing, IL-17, TNF with IFN-γ produced only with *Mtb* lysate. Though we had a significant increase in CD4$^+$ and CD8$^+$ T cells this did not translate into changes or improved lung pathology or bacterial burdens. Therefore, despite enhanced T cells, other factors or cell population play a role in *Mtb* infection.

It would appear IL-4Rα on Foxp3 T cells may not be contributing to controlling *Mtb* during the early and late phase of infections but affect the effector T cells similarly to *Lm* infection. We suggestion this discrepancy between these two models might be due in part that; in the *Lm* model, there was a significant increase in neutrophils, and as discussed above, neutrophils are known to play a beneficial role during early *Lm* infection (Conlan 1997), conversely, increase neutrophils have been shown to be detrimental during *Mtb* infection owing to the fact that there are the first cells to migrate to the site of infection (Eruslanov *et al.* 2005). Also, CD8$^+$ cytotoxic T cells play an essential and predominant role during *Lm* infection (Lara-Tejero & Pamer 2004; Condotta *et al.* 2012) due to the recognition of specific epitopes in MHC-1 cytosolic presentation(Shen *et al.* 1998). On the other hand, CD8$^+$T cells play a role in *Mtb* infection but are not indispensable in the same light as CD4$^+$ T cells (Mogues *et al.* 2001).

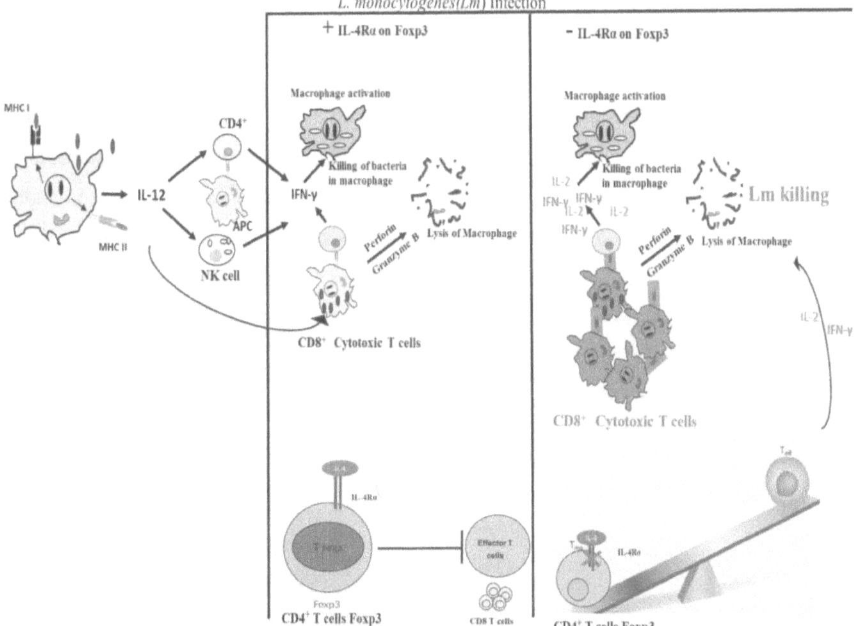

Figure 4.1 Proposed model on gain/loss of IL-4Rα on CD4$^+$ T Foxp3 during *Lm* infection

During infection, macrophages phagocytise the *Lm* and produce IL-12 that recruits other myeloid cells and present it to naive CD4$^+$ T cells to produce IFN-γ and other cytokines including IL-2 Presence of IL-4Rα on CD4 T Foxp3 maintains Foxp3 T reg during *Lm* infection. However, loss of IL-4Rα leads to the loss of a percentage of Foxp3 T reg thereby shifting the balance towards a more effector T cell. Effector T cells are characterised by the presence of T-bet transcriptional factor hallmark of Th-1 responses. Th-1 secrete IFN-γ and IL-4 that probable activates macrophages to kill *Lm* during infection.

In conclusion, several studies had demonstrated the detrimental role of IL-4/IL-4Rα signalling in the promotion of Th-1 immune responses. To our knowledge, no study has described a cell-specific deletion of IL-4Rα during *Lm*. A Foxp3 T cell-deficient of IL-4Rα (Foxp3^{cre}IL-4Rα$^{-/lox}$) allowed us to investigate an important role of the stability of CD4 Foxp3 T reg in the absence of IL-4Rα during *Lm* infection. Infection of Foxp3^{cre}IL-4Rα$^{-/lox}$ mice with *Lm* led to the loss of the quality, thereby, tilting the CD4 T cell effector balance to more effector phenotype. Optimal immunity depends on a robust and clonal expansion of effector T cell function that renders the cells to secrete cytokines that mount a rapid response to pathogens during infection (Zhou *et al.* 2009).

These led to the production of pro-inflammatory cytokines, including IFN-γ which are essential for *Lm* clearance. Strikingly, in $CD4^+CD25^+$ T cell sorted from $Foxp3^{cre}IL\text{-}4R\alpha^{-/lox}$ mice confirmed an important role of the suppressive nature of T reg through the secretion of IL-10. In *Mtb* infection, we did not observe any differences in bacterial burden and histopathology. Future study will address whether a virulent strain of *Mtb* affects the outcome in this mouse model.However, the CD4 T effector balance was significantly altered in the absence of IL-4Rα, similarly to *Lm* infection. Together we demonstrate a novel role of IL-4Rα signalling during Th1 models of Listeriosis and tuberculosis.

REFERENCES

Adalid-Peralta, L., Fragoso, G., Fleury, A. & Sciutto, E. (2011) Mechanisms Underlying the Induction of Regulatory T cells and Its Relevance in the Adaptive Immune Response in Parasitic Infections. *International Journal of Biological Sciences* **7**: 1412–1426.

Akira, S., Uematsu, S. & Takeuchi, O. (2006) Pathogen Recognition and Innate Immunity. *Cell* **124**: 783–801.

Andersson, Å., Dai, W. J., Santo, J. P. D. & Brombacher, F. (1998) Early IFN-γ Production and Innate Immunity During Listeria monocytogenes Infection in the Absence of NK Cells. *The Journal of Immunology* **161**: 5600–5606.

Annunziato, F. & Romagnani, S. (2009) Heterogeneity of human effector CD4+T cells. *Arthritis Research & Therapy* **11**: 257.

Aoshi, T., Zinselmeyer, B. H., Konjufca, V., Lynch, J. N., Zhang, X., Koide, Y. & Miller, M. J. (2008) Bacterial Entry to the Splenic White Pulp Initiates Antigen Presentation to CD8+ T Cells. *Immunity* **29**: 476–486.

Arenas-Ramirez, N., Woytschak, J. & Boyman, O. (2015) Interleukin-2: Biology, Design and Application. *Trends in Immunology* **36**: 763–777.

Arun, K. V., Talwar, A. & Kumar, T. S. S. (2011) T-helper cells in the etiopathogenesis of periodontal disease: A mini review. *Journal of Indian Society of Periodontology* **15**: 4.

Aziz, N. A., Nono, J. K., Mpotje, T. & Brombacher, F. (2018) The Foxp3+ regulatory T-cell population requires IL-4Rα signaling to control inflammation during helminth infections. *PLOS Biology* **16**: e2005850.

Bancroft, G. J., Schreiber, R. D. & Unanue, E. R. (1991) Natural immunity: a T-cell-independent pathway of macrophage activation, defined in the scid mouse. *Immunological Reviews* **124**: 5–24.

Barberis, I., Bragazzi, N. L., Galluzzo, L. & Martini, M. (2017) The history of tuberculosis: from the first historical records to the isolation of Koch's bacillus. *Journal of Preventive Medicine and Hygiene* **58**: E9–E12.

Barbosa, B. F., Lopes-Maria, J. B., Gomes, A. O., Angeloni, M. B., Castro, A. S., Franco, P. S., Fermino, M. L., Roque-Barreira, M. C., Ietta, F., Martins-Filho, O. A., Silva, D. A. O., Mineo, J. R. & Ferro, E. A. V. (2015) IL10, TGF Beta1, and IFN Gamma Modulate Intracellular Signaling Pathways and Cytokine Production to Control Toxoplasma gondii Infection in BeWo Trophoblast Cells1. *Biology of Reproduction* **92**.

Bean, A. G., Roach, D. R., Briscoe, H., France, M. P., Korner, H., Sedgwick, J. D. & Britton, W. J. (1999) Structural deficiencies in granuloma formation in TNF gene-targeted mice underlie the heightened susceptibility to aerosol Mycobacterium tuberculosis infection, which is not compensated for by lymphotoxin. *Journal of Immunology (Baltimore, Md.: 1950)* **162**: 3504–3511.

Behr, M. A., Edelstein, P. H. & Ramakrishnan, L. (2018) Revisiting the timetable of tuberculosis. *BMJ* **362**: k2738.

Belkaid, Y., Piccirillo, C. A., Mendez, S., Shevach, E. M. & Sacks, D. L. (2002) CD4+CD25+ regulatory T cells control Leishmania major persistence and immunity. *Nature* **420**: 502–507.

Bending, D., De la Peña, H., Veldhoen, M., Phillips, J. M., Uyttenhove, C., Stockinger, B. & Cooke, A. (2009) Highly purified Th17 cells from BDC2.5NOD mice convert into Th1-like cells in NOD/SCID recipient mice. *The Journal of Clinical Investigation* **119**: 565–572.

Benmerzoug, S., Marinho, F. V., Rose, S., Mackowiak, C., Gosset, D., Sedda, D., Poisson, E., Uyttenhove, C., Van Snick, J., Jacobs, M., Garcia, I., Ryffel, B. & Quesniaux, V. F. J. (2018) GM-CSF targeted immunomodulation affects host response to M. tuberculosis infection. *Scientific Reports* **8**: 8652.

Berche, P., Gaillard, J. L. & Sansonetti, P. J. (1987) Intracellular growth of Listeria monocytogenes as a prerequisite for in vivo induction of T cell-mediated immunity. *The Journal of Immunology* **138**: 2266–2271.

Berry, M. P. R., Graham, C. M., McNab, F. W., Xu, Z., Bloch, S. A. A., Oni, T., Wilkinson, K. A., Banchereau, R., Skinner, J., Wilkinson, R. J., Quinn, C., Blankenship, D., Dhawan, R., Cush, J. J., Mejias, A., Ramilo, O., Kon, O. M., Pascual, V., Banchereau, J., Chaussabel, D. & O'Garra, A. (2010) An interferon-inducible neutrophil-driven blood transcriptional signature in human tuberculosis. *Nature* **466**: 973.

Bettelli, E., Oukka, M. & Kuchroo, V. K. (2007) TH-17 cells in the circle of immunity and autoimmunity. *Nature Immunology* **8**: 345.

Bhattacharya, P., Thiruppathi, M., Elshabrawy, H. A., Alharshawi, K., Kumar, P. & Prabhakar, B. S. (2015) GM-CSF: An Immune Modulatory Cytokine that can Suppress Autoimmunity. *Cytokine* **75**: 261–271.

Biedermann, T., Zimmermann, S., Himmelrich, H., Gumy, A., Egeter, O., Sakrauski, A. K., Seegmüller, I., Voigt, H., Launois, P., Levine, A. D., Wagner, H., Heeg, K., Louis, J. A. & Röcken, M. (2001) IL-4 instructs TH1 responses and resistance to Leishmania major in susceptible BALB/c mice. *Nature Immunology* **2**: 1054–1060.

Bielecki, J., Youngman, P., Connelly, P. & Portnoy, D. A. (1990) Bacillus subtilis expressing a haemolysin gene from Listeria monocytogenes can grow in mammalian cells. *Nature* **345**: 175–176.

Bissonnette, R. P., Echeverri, F., Mahboubi, A. & Green, D. R. (1992) Apoptotic cell death induced by c-myc is inhibited by bcl-2. *Nature* **359**: 552–554.

Bloom, C. I., Graham, C. M., Berry, M. P. R., Rozakeas, F., Redford, P. S., Wang, Y., Xu, Z., Wilkinson, K. A., Wilkinson, R. J., Kendrick, Y., Devouassoux, G., Ferry, T., Miyara, M., Bouvry, D., Valeyre, D., Dominique, V., Gorochov, G., Blankenship, D., Saadatian, M., Vanhems, P., Beynon, H., Vancheeswaran, R., Wickremasinghe, M., Chaussabel,

D., Banchereau, J., Pascual, V., Ho, L.-P., Lipman, M. & O'Garra, A. (2013) Transcriptional blood signatures distinguish pulmonary tuberculosis, pulmonary sarcoidosis, pneumonias and lung cancers. *PloS One* **8**: e70630.

Bluestone, J. A. & Tang, Q. (2005) How do CD4+CD25+ regulatory T cells control autoimmunity? *Current Opinion in Immunology* **17**: 638–642.

Bonazzi, M., Veiga, E., Pizarro-Cerdá, J. & Cossart, P. (2008) Successive post-translational modifications of E-cadherin are required for InlA-mediated internalization of Listeria monocytogenes. *Cellular Microbiology* **10**: 2208–2222.

Brombacher, F., Dorfmüller, A., Magram, J., Dai, W. J., Köhler, G., Wunderlin, A., Palmer-Lehmann, K., Gately, M. K. & Alber, G. (1999) IL-12 is dispensable for innate and adaptive immunity against low doses of Listeria monocytogenes. *International Immunology* **11**: 325–332.

Bruns, H., Meinken, C., Schauenberg, P., Härter, G., Kern, P., Modlin, R. L., Antoni, C. & Stenger, S. (2009) Anti-TNF immunotherapy reduces CD8+ T cell-mediated antimicrobial activity against Mycobacterium tuberculosis in humans. *The Journal of Clinical Investigation* **119**: 1167–1177.

Buccheri, S., Reljic, R., Caccamo, N., Ivanyi, J., Singh, M., Salerno, A. & Dieli, F. (2007) IL-4 depletion enhances host resistance and passive IgA protection against tuberculosis infection in BALB/c mice. *European Journal of Immunology* **37**: 729–737.

Buchmeier, N. A. & Schreiber, R. D. (1985) Requirement of endogenous interferon-gamma production for resolution of Listeria monocytogenes infection. *Proceedings of the National Academy of Sciences* **82**: 7404.

Burl, S., Hill, P. C., Jeffries, D. J., Holland, M. J., Fox, A., Lugos, M. D., Adegbola, R. A., Rook, G. A., Zumla, A., McAdam, K. P. W. J. & Brookes, R. H. (2007) FOXP3 gene expression in a tuberculosis case contact study. *Clinical and Experimental Immunology* **149**: 117–122.

Busch, D. H., Pilip, I. M., Vijh, S. & Pamer, E. G. (1998) Coordinate Regulation of Complex T Cell Populations Responding to Bacterial Infection. *Immunity* **8**: 353–362.

Campbell, D. J. & Koch, M. A. (2011) Phenotypical and functional specialization of FOXP3+ regulatory T cells. *Nature Reviews Immunology* **11**: 119.

Cao, Y., Brombacher, F., Tunyogi-Csapo, M., Glant, T. T. & Finnegan, A. (2007) Interleukin-4 regulates proteoglycan-induced arthritis by specifically suppressing the innate immune response. *Arthritis and Rheumatism* **56**: 861–870.

Carr, K. D., Sieve, A. N., Indramohan, M., Break, T. J., Lee, S. & Berg, R. E. (2011) Specific depletion reveals a novel role for neutrophil-mediated protection in the liver during Listeria monocytogenes infection. *European journal of immunology* **41**: 2666–2676.

Carrero, J. A., Calderon, B. & Unanue, E. R. (2004) Listeriolysin O from <em>Listeria monocytogenes</em> Is a Lymphocyte Apoptogenic Molecule. *The Journal of Immunology* **172**: 4866.

Chackerian, A. A., Alt, J. M., Perera, T. V., Dascher, C. C. & Behar, S. M. (2002) Dissemination of Mycobacterium tuberculosis is influenced by host factors and precedes the initiation of T-cell immunity. *Infection and Immunity* **70**: 4501–4509.

Chai, J.-G., Coe, D., Chen, D., Simpson, E., Dyson, J. & Scott, D. (2008) In Vitro Expansion Improves In Vivo Regulation by CD4$^+$CD25$^+$ Regulatory T Cells. *The Journal of Immunology* **180**: 858.

Chan, J., Xing, Y., Magliozzo, R. S. & Bloom, B. R. (1992) Killing of virulent Mycobacterium tuberculosis by reactive nitrogen intermediates produced by activated murine macrophages. *The Journal of Experimental Medicine* **175**: 1111–1122.

Chen, X., Zhou, B., Li, M., Deng, Q., Wu, X., Le, X., Wu, C., Larmonier, N., Zhang, W., Zhang, H., Wang, H. & Katsanis, E. (2007) CD4(+)CD25(+)FoxP3(+) regulatory T cells suppress Mycobacterium tuberculosis immunity in patients with active disease. *Clinical Immunology (Orlando, Fla.)* **123**: 50–59.

Classen, A., Lloberas, J. & Celada, A. (2009) Macrophage activation: classical versus alternative. *Methods in Molecular Biology (Clifton, N.J.)* **531**: 29–43.

Cliff, J. M., Lee, J.-S., Constantinou, N., Cho, J.-E., Clark, T. G., Ronacher, K., King, E. C., Lukey, P. T., Duncan, K., Van Helden, P. D., Walzl, G. & Dockrell, H. M. (2013) Distinct phases of blood gene expression pattern through tuberculosis treatment reflect modulation of the humoral immune response. *The Journal of Infectious Diseases* **207**: 18–29.

Condotta, S. A., Richer, M. J., Badovinac, V. P. & Harty, J. T. (2012) Probing CD8 T cell responses with Listeria monocytogenes infection. *Advances in Immunology* **113**: 51–80.

Conlan, J. W. (1997) Critical roles of neutrophils in host defense against experimental systemic infections of mice by Listeria monocytogenes, Salmonella typhimurium, and Yersinia enterocolitica. *Infection and Immunity* **65**: 630–635.

Conlan, J. W. & North, R. J. (1994) Neutrophils are essential for early anti-Listeria defense in the liver, but not in the spleen or peritoneal cavity, as revealed by a granulocyte-depleting monoclonal antibody. *The Journal of Experimental Medicine* **179**: 259.

Cooper, A. M. (2009) Cell-Mediated Immune Responses in Tuberculosis. *Annual Review of Immunology* **27**: 393–422.

Cooper, A. M., Mayer-Barber, K. D. & Sher, A. (2011) Role of innate cytokines in mycobacterial infection. *Mucosal Immunology* **4**: 252.

Cosmi, L., Liotta, F., Angeli, R., Mazzinghi, B., Santarlasci, V., Manetti, R., Lasagni, L., Vanini, V., Romagnani, P., Maggi, E., Annunziato, F. & Romagnani, S. (2004) Th2 cells are less susceptible than Th1 cells to the suppressive activity of CD25+ regulatory thymocytes because of their responsiveness to different cytokines. *Blood* **103**: 3117–3121.

Cossart, P. & Helenius, A. (2014) Endocytosis of viruses and bacteria. *Cold Spring Harbor Perspectives in Biology* **6**.

Cossart, P., Vicente, M. F., Mengaud, J., Baquero, F., Perez-Diaz, J. C. & Berche, P. (1989) Listeriolysin O is essential for virulence of Listeria monocytogenes: direct evidence obtained by gene complementation. *Infection and Immunity* **57**: 3629–3636.

Cousens, L. P. & Wing, E. J. (2000) Innate defenses in the liver during Listeria infection. *Immunological Reviews* **174**: 150–159.

van Crevel, R., Karyadi, E., Preyers, F., Leenders, M., Kullberg, B.-J., Nelwan, R. H. H. & van der Meer, J. W. M. (2000) Increased Production of Interleukin 4 by CD4+ and CD8+ T Cells from Patients with Tuberculosis Is Related to the Presence of Pulmonary Cavities. *The Journal of Infectious Diseases* **181**: 1194–1197.

Cruz, A., Fraga, A. G., Fountain, J. J., Rangel-Moreno, J., Torrado, E., Saraiva, M., Pereira, D. R., Randall, T. D., Pedrosa, J., Cooper, A. M. & Castro, A. G. (2010) Pathological role of interleukin 17 in mice subjected to repeated BCG vaccination after infection with Mycobacterium tuberculosis. *The Journal of experimental medicine* **207**: 1609–1616.

Curtsinger, J. M., Lins, D. C. & Mescher, M. F. (2003) Signal 3 determines tolerance versus full activation of naive CD8 T cells: dissociating proliferation and development of effector function. *The Journal of Experimental Medicine* **197**: 1141–1151.

Curtsinger, J. M., Valenzuela, J. O., Agarwal, P., Lins, D. & Mescher, M. F. (2005) Type I IFNs provide a third signal to CD8 T cells to stimulate clonal expansion and differentiation. *Journal of Immunology (Baltimore, Md.: 1950)* **174**: 4465–4469.

Czuprynski, C. J. & Brown, J. F. (1990) Effects of purified anti-Lyt-2 mAb treatment on murine listeriosis: comparative roles of Lyt-2+ and L3T4+ cells in resistance to primary and secondary infection, delayed-type hypersensitivity and adoptive transfer of resistance. *Immunology* **71**: 107–112.

Czuprynski, C. J., Brown, J. F., Maroushek, N., Wagner, R. D. & Steinberg, H. (1994) Administration of anti-granulocyte mAb RB6-8C5 impairs the resistance of mice to Listeria monocytogenes infection. *The Journal of Immunology* **152**: 1836.

Dai, W. J., Bartens, W., Köhler, G., Hufnagel, M., Kopf, M. & Brombacher, F. (1997) Impaired macrophage listericidal and cytokine activities are responsible for the rapid death of Listeria monocytogenes-infected IFN-gamma receptor-deficient mice. *The Journal of Immunology* **158**: 5297–5304.

Daniel, V. S. & Daniel, T. M. (1999) Old Testament biblical references to tuberculosis. *Clinical Infectious Diseases: An Official Publication of the Infectious Diseases Society of America* **29**: 1557–1558.

Dardalhon, V., Awasthi, A., Kwon, H., Galileos, G., Gao, W., Sobel, R. A., Mitsdoerffer, M., Strom, T. B., Elyaman, W., Ho, I.-C., Khoury, S., Oukka, M. & Kuchroo, V. K. (2008) Interleukin 4 inhibits TGF-β-induced-Foxp3+T cells and generates, in combination with TGF-β, Foxp3− effector T cells that produce interleukins 9 and 10. *Nature immunology* **9**: 1347–1355.

Davidson, S., Maini, M. K. & Wack, A. (2015) Disease-Promoting Effects of Type I Interferons in Viral, Bacterial, and Coinfections. *Journal of Interferon & Cytokine Research* **35**: 252–264.

Dawany, N., Showe, L. C., Kossenkov, A. V., Chang, C., Ive, P., Conradie, F., Stevens, W., Sanne, I., Azzoni, L. & Montaner, L. J. (2014) Identification of a 251 gene expression signature that can accurately detect M. tuberculosis in patients with and without HIV co-infection. *PloS One* **9**: e89925.

D'Cruz, L. M., Rubinstein, M. P. & Goldrath, A. W. (2009) Surviving the crash: transitioning from effector to memory CD8+ T cell. *Seminars in Immunology* **21**: 92–98.

Dempsey, P. W., Vaidya, S. A. & Cheng, G. (2003) The Art of War: Innate and adaptive immune responses. *Cellular and Molecular Life Sciences CMLS* **60**: 2604–2621.

Desai, A. N., Anyoha, A., Madoff, L. C. & Lassmann, B. (2019) Changing epidemiology of Listeria monocytogenes outbreaks, sporadic cases, and recalls globally: A review of ProMED reports from 1996 to 2018. *International journal of infectious diseases : IJID : official publication of the International Society for Infectious Diseases* **84**: 48–53.

Dewals, B., Hoving, J. C., Leeto, M., Marillier, R. G., Govender, U., Cutler, A. J., Horsnell, W. G. C. & Brombacher, F. (2009) IL-4Rα Responsiveness of Non-CD4 T Cells Contributes to Resistance in Schistosoma mansoni Infection in Pan-T Cell-Specific IL-4Rα-Deficient Mice. *The American Journal of Pathology* **175**: 706–716.

Dheda, K., Chang, J.-S., Huggett, J. F., Kim, L. U., Johnson, M. A., Zumla, A. & Rook, G. A. W. (2007) The stability of mRNA encoding IL-4 is increased in pulmonary tuberculosis, while stability of mRNA encoding the antagonistic splice variant, IL-4delta2, is not. *Tuberculosis (Edinburgh, Scotland)* **87**: 237–241.

Dinarello, C. A. (2007) Historical Review of Cytokines. *European journal of immunology* **37**: S34–S45.

van Dissel, J. T., Stikkelbroeck, J. J., Michel, B. C., van den Barselaar, M. T., Leijh, P. C. & van Furth, R. (1987) Inability of recombinant interferon-gamma to activate the antibacterial activity of mouse peritoneal macrophages against Listeria monocytogenes and Salmonella typhimurium. *The Journal of Immunology* **139**: 1673.

Dolina, J. S. & Schoenberger, S. P. (2017*a*) Toll-like receptor 9 is required for the maintenance of CD25⁺FoxP3⁺CD4⁺ T$_{reg}$ cells during <em>Listeria monocytogenes</em> infection. *The Journal of Immunology* **198**: 151.9.

Dolina, J. S. & Schoenberger, S. P. (2017*b*) Toll-like receptor 9 is required for the maintenance of CD25+FoxP3+CD4+ Treg cells during Listeria monocytogenes infection. *The Journal of Immunology* **198**: 151.9-151.9.

Dowling, M. R., Kan, A., Heinzel, S., Marchingo, J. M., Hodgkin, P. D. & Hawkins, E. D. (2018) Regulatory T Cells Suppress Effector T Cell Proliferation by Limiting Division Destiny. *Frontiers in Immunology* **9**.

Dunne, D. W., Resnick, D., Greenberg, J., Krieger, M. & Joiner, K. A. (1994) The type I macrophage scavenger receptor binds to gram-positive bacteria and recognizes lipoteichoic acid. *Proceedings of the National Academy of Sciences of the United States of America* **91**: 1863–1867.

Durant, L., Watford, W. T., Ramos, H. L., Laurence, A., Vahedi, G., Wei, L., Takahashi1, H., Sun, H.-W., Kanno, Y., Powrie, F. & O'Shea, J. J. (2010) Diverse Targets of the Transcription Factor STAT3 Contribute to T Cell Pathogenicity and Homeostasis. *Immunity* **32**: 605–615.

Edelson, B. T. & Unanue, E. R. (2001) Intracellular Antibody Neutralizes Listeria Growth. *Immunity* **14**: 503–512.

Edelson, B. T., Bradstreet, T. R., Hildner, K., Carrero, J. A., Frederick, K. E., Kc, W., Belizaire, R., Aoshi, T., Schreiber, R. D., Miller, M. J., Murphy, T. L., Unanue, E. R. & Murphy, K. M. (2011*a*) CD8α(+) dendritic cells are an obligate cellular entry point for productive infection by Listeria monocytogenes. *Immunity* **35**: 236–248.

Edelson, B. T., Bradstreet, T. R., Hildner, K., Carrero, J. A., Frederick, K. E., KC, W., Belizaire, R., Aoshi, T., Schreiber, R. D., Miller, M. J., Murphy, T. L., Unanue, E. R. & Murphy, K. M. (2011*b*) CD8α+ Dendritic Cells Are an Obligate Cellular Entry Point for Productive Infection by Listeria monocytogenes. *Immunity* **35**: 236–248.

Eisenstein, E. M. & Williams, C. B. (2009) The T reg /Th17 Cell Balance: A New Paradigm for Autoimmunity. *Pediatric Research* **65**: 26–31.

Emoto, Y., Emoto, M. & Kaufmann, S. H. (1997) Transient control of interleukin-4-producing natural killer T cells in the livers of Listeria monocytogenes-infected mice by interleukin-12. *Infection and Immunity* **65**: 5003–5009.

Ertelt, J. M., Rowe, J. H., Johanns, T. M., Lai, J. C., McLachlan, J. B. & Way, S. S. (2009*a*) Selective Priming and Expansion of Antigen-Specific Foxp3⁻CD4⁺ T Cells during <em>Listeria monocytogenes</em> Infection. *The Journal of Immunology* **182**: 3032.

Ertelt, J. M., Rowe, J. H., Johanns, T. M., Lai, J. C., McLachlan, J. B. & Way, S. S. (2009*b*) Selective Priming and Expansion of Antigen-Specific Foxp3−CD4+ T Cells during Listeria monocytogenes Infection. *The Journal of Immunology* **182**: 3032.

Ertelt, J. M., Rowe, J. H., Mysz, M. A., Singh, C., Roychowdhury, M., Aguilera, M. N. & Way, S. S. (2011) Foxp3+ regulatory T cells impede the priming of protective CD8+ T cells. *Journal of immunology (Baltimore, Md. : 1950)* **187**: 2569–2577.

Eruslanov, E. B., Lyadova, I. V., Kondratieva, T. K., Majorov, K. B., Scheglov, I. V., Orlova, M. O. & Apt, A. S. (2005*a*) Neutrophil Responses to <em>Mycobacterium tuberculosis</em> Infection in Genetically Susceptible and Resistant Mice. *Infection and Immunity* **73**: 1744.

Eruslanov, E. B., Lyadova, I. V., Kondratieva, T. K., Majorov, K. B., Scheglov, I. V., Orlova, M. O. & Apt, A. S. (2005*b*) Neutrophil Responses to Mycobacterium tuberculosis Infection in Genetically Susceptible and Resistant Mice. *Infection and Immunity* **73**: 1744.

Ferraris, D. M., Gherardi, E., Di, Y., Heinz, D. W. & Niemann, H. H. (2010) Ligand-mediated dimerization of the Met receptor tyrosine kinase by the bacterial invasion protein InlB. *Journal of Molecular Biology* **395**: 522–532.

Ferreira, V., Wiedmann, M., Teixeira, P. & Stasiewicz, M. J. (2014) Listeria monocytogenes persistence in food-associated environments: epidemiology, strain characteristics, and implications for public health. *Journal of Food Protection* **77**: 150–170.

Finelli, A., Kerksiek, K. M., Allen, S. E., Marshall, N., Mercado, R., Pilip, I., Busch, D. H. & Pamer, E. G. (1999) MHC class I restricted T cell responses to Listeria monocytogenes, an intracellular bacterial pathogen. *Immunologic Research* **19**: 211–223.

Flynn, J., Chan, J. & Lin, P. (2011) Macrophages and control of granulomatous inflammation in tuberculosis. *Mucosal Immunology* **4**: 271–278.

Fontenot, J. D., Rasmussen, J. P., Williams, L. M., Dooley, J. L., Farr, A. G. & Rudensky, A. Y. (2005) Regulatory T cell lineage specification by the forkhead transcription factor foxp3. *Immunity* **22**: 329–341.

Gaillard, J. L., Berche, P., Frehel, C., Gouin, E. & Cossart, P. (1991) Entry of L. monocytogenes into cells is mediated by internalin, a repeat protein reminiscent of surface antigens from gram-positive cocci. *Cell* **65**: 1127–1141.

Garrison, F. H. (1921) *An introduction to the history of medicine: with medical chronology, suggestions for study and bibliographic data*. Philadelphia: Saunders.

Geldmacher, C., Zumla, A. & Hoelscher, M. (2012) Interaction between HIV and Mycobacterium tuberculosis: HIV-1-induced CD4 T-cell depletion and the development of active tuberculosis. *Current opinion in HIV and AIDS* **7**: 268–275.

Glomski, I. J., Gedde, M. M., Tsang, A. W., Swanson, J. A. & Portnoy, D. A. (2002) The Listeria monocytogenes hemolysin has an acidic pH optimum to compartmentalize activity and prevent damage to infected host cells. *The Journal of Cell Biology* **156**: 1029–1038.

Gopal, R., Lin, Y., Obermajer, N., Slight, S., Nuthalapati, N., Ahmed, M., Kalinski, P. & Khader, S. A. (2012) IL-23-dependent IL-17 drives Th1-cell responses following Mycobacterium bovis BCG vaccination. *European Journal of Immunology* **42**: 364–373.

Gordon, S. (2003) Alternative activation of macrophages. *Nature Reviews. Immunology* **3**: 23–35.

Goulet, V., King, L. A., Vaillant, V. & de Valk, H. (2013) What is the incubation period for listeriosis? *BMC Infectious Diseases* **13**: 11.

Graw, F., Weber, K. S., Allen, P. M. & Perelson, A. S. (2012) Dynamics of CD4(+) T cell responses against Listeria monocytogenes. *Journal of immunology (Baltimore, Md. : 1950)* **189**: 5250–5256.

Green, A. M., Mattila, J. T., Bigbee, C. L., Bongers, K. S., Lin, P. L. & Flynn, J. L. (2010) CD4(+) regulatory T cells in a cynomolgus macaque model of Mycobacterium tuberculosis infection. *The Journal of Infectious Diseases* **202**: 533–541.

Greenberg, J. W., Fischer, W. & Joiner, K. A. (1996) Influence of lipoteichoic acid structure on recognition by the macrophage scavenger receptor. *Infection and Immunity* **64**: 3318–3325.

Gregory, S. H. & Wing, E. J. (2002) Neutrophil-Kupffer cell interaction: a critical component of host defenses to systemic bacterial infections. *Journal of Leukocyte Biology* **72**: 239–248.

Guler, R., Parihar, S. P., Savvi, S., Logan, E., Schwegmann, A., Roy, S., Nieuwenhuizen, N. E., Ozturk, M., Schmeier, S., Suzuki, H. & Brombacher, F. (2015) IL-4Rα-Dependent Alternative Activation of Macrophages Is Not Decisive for Mycobacterium tuberculosis Pathology and Bacterial Burden in Mice. *PLoS ONE* **10**.

Gunn, G. R., Zubair, A., Peters, C., Pan, Z. K., Wu, T. C. & Paterson, Y. (2001) Two Listeria monocytogenes vaccine vectors that express different molecular forms of human papilloma virus-16 (HPV-16) E7 induce qualitatively different T cell immunity that correlates with their ability to induce regression of established tumors immortalized by HPV-16. *Journal of Immunology (Baltimore, Md.: 1950)* **167**: 6471–6479.

Gutierrez, M. C., Brisse, S., Brosch, R., Fabre, M., Omaïs, B., Marmiesse, M., Supply, P. & Vincent, V. (2005) Ancient origin and gene mosaicism of the progenitor of Mycobacterium tuberculosis. *PLoS pathogens* **1**: e5.

Gutierrez, M. G., Master, S. S., Singh, S. B., Taylor, G. A., Colombo, M. I. & Deretic, V. (2004) Autophagy is a defense mechanism inhibiting BCG and Mycobacterium tuberculosis survival in infected macrophages. *Cell* **119**: 753–766.

Guyot-Revol, V., Innes, J. A., Hackforth, S., Hinks, T. & Lalvani, A. (2006) Regulatory T cells are expanded in blood and disease sites in patients with tuberculosis. *American Journal of Respiratory and Critical Care Medicine* **173**: 803–810.

Haak-Frendscho, M., Brown, J. F., Iizawa, Y., Wagner, R. D. & Czuprynski, C. J. (1992) Administration of anti-IL-4 monoclonal antibody 11B11 increases the resistance of mice to Listeria monocytogenes infection. *The Journal of Immunology* **148**: 3978.

Hale, J. S. & Ahmed, R. (2015) Memory T Follicular Helper CD4 T Cells. *Frontiers in Immunology* **6**: 16.

Hamon, M., Bierne, H. & Cossart, P. (2006) Listeria monocytogenes: a multifaceted model. *Nature Reviews. Microbiology* **4**: 423–434.

Hansmann, L., Schmidl, C., Kett, J., Steger, L., Andreesen, R., Hoffmann, P., Rehli, M. & Edinger, M. (2012) Dominant Th2 Differentiation of Human Regulatory T Cells upon Loss of FOXP3 Expression. *The Journal of Immunology* **188**: 1275–1282.

Haque, A., Best, S. E., Amante, F. H., Mustafah, S., Desbarrieres, L., de Labastida, F., Sparwasser, T., Hill, G. R. & Engwerda, C. R. (2010) CD4+ Natural Regulatory T Cells Prevent Experimental Cerebral Malaria via CTLA-4 When Expanded In Vivo. *PLoS Pathogens* **6**.

Harris, J., De Haro, S. A., Master, S. S., Keane, J., Roberts, E. A., Delgado, M. & Deretic, V. (2007) T helper 2 cytokines inhibit autophagic control of intracellular Mycobacterium tuberculosis. *Immunity* **27**: 505–517.

Hart, T. K., Blackburn, M. N., Brigham-Burke, M., Dede, K., Al-Mahdi, N., Zia-Amirhosseini, P. & Cook, R. M. (2002) Preclinical efficacy and safety of pascolizumab (SB 240683): a humanized anti-interleukin-4 antibody with therapeutic potential in asthma. *Clinical and Experimental Immunology* **130**: 93–100.

Harty, J. T. & Badovinac, V. P. (2002) Influence of effector molecules on the CD8+ T cell response to infection. *Current Opinion in Immunology* **14**: 360–365.

Harty, J. T., Lenz, L. L. & Bevan, M. J. (1996) Primary and secondary immune responses to Listeria monocytogenes. *Current opinion in immunology* **8**: 526–530.

Hayman, J. (1984) MYCOBACTERIUM ULCERANS: AN INFECTION FROM JURASSIC TIME? *Originally published as Volume 2, Issue 8410* **324**: 1015–1016.

Heitmann, L., Dar, M. A., Schreiber, T., Erdmann, H., Behrends, J., Mckenzie, A. N., Brombacher, F., Ehlers, S. & Hölscher, C. (2014) The IL-13/IL-4Rα axis is involved in tuberculosis-associated pathology. *The Journal of Pathology* **234**: 338–350.

Helwani, F. M., Kovacs, E. M., Paterson, A. D., Verma, S., Ali, R. G., Fanning, A. S., Weed, S. A. & Yap, A. S. (2004) Cortactin is necessary for E-cadherin-mediated contact formation and actin reorganization. *The Journal of Cell Biology* **164**: 899–910.

Hernandez-Pando, R., Aguilar, D., Hernandez, M. L. G., Orozco, H. & Rook, G. (2004) Pulmonary tuberculosis in BALB/c mice with non-functional IL-4 genes: changes in the inflammatory effects of TNF-alpha and in the regulation of fibrosis. *European Journal of Immunology* **34**: 174–183.

Hill, J. A., Feuerer, M., Tash, K., Haxhinasto, S., Perez, J., Melamed, R., Mathis, D. & Benoist, C. (2007) Foxp3 Transcription-Factor-Dependent and -Independent Regulation of the Regulatory T Cell Transcriptional Signature. *Immunity* **27**: 786–800.

Hiltbold, E. M. & Ziegler, H. K. (1993) Mechanisms of processing and presentation of the antigens of Listeria monocytogenes. *Infectious Agents and Disease* **2**: 314–323.

Hoge, J., Yan, I., Jänner, N., Schumacher, V., Chalaris, A., Steinmetz, O. M., Engel, D. R., Scheller, J., Rose-John, S. & Mittrücker, H.-W. (2013) IL-6 Controls the Innate Immune Response against Listeria monocytogenes via Classical IL-6 Signaling. *The Journal of Immunology* **190**: 703–711.

Hölscher, C., Arendse, B., Schwegmann, A., Myburgh, E. & Brombacher, F. (2006) Impairment of alternative macrophage activation delays cutaneous leishmaniasis in nonhealing BALB/c mice. *Journal of Immunology (Baltimore, Md.: 1950)* **176**: 1115–1121.

Hori, S., Nomura, T. & Sakaguchi, S. (2003) Control of regulatory T cell development by the transcription factor Foxp3. *Science (New York, N.Y.)* **299**: 1057–1061.

Horsburgh, C. R. & Rubin, E. J. (2011) Clinical practice. Latent tuberculosis infection in the United States. *The New England Journal of Medicine* **364**: 1441–1448.

Houston, M. (1999) The White Death: A History of Tuberculosis. *BMJ : British Medical Journal* **318**: 1705.

Hoving, J. C., Kirstein, F., Nieuwenhuizen, N. E., Fick, L. C. E., Hobeika, E., Reth, M. & Brombacher, F. (2012) B Cells That Produce Immunoglobulin E Mediate Colitis in BALB/c Mice. *Gastroenterology* **142**: 96–108.

Hsieh, C., Macatonia, S., Tripp, C., Wolf, S., O'Garra, A. & Murphy, K. (1993) Development of TH1 CD4+ T cells through IL-12 produced by Listeria-induced macrophages. *Science* **260**: 547.

Hurdayal, R., Nieuwenhuizen, N. E., Revaz-Breton, M., Smith, L., Hoving, J. C., Parihar, S. P., Reizis, B. & Brombacher, F. (2013) Deletion of IL-4 Receptor Alpha on Dendritic Cells Renders BALB/c Mice Hypersusceptible to Leishmania major Infection. *PLOS Pathogens* **9**: e1003699.

Hussain, S. F. & Paterson, Y. (2004) CD4+CD25+ regulatory T cells that secrete TGFbeta and IL-10 are preferentially induced by a vaccine vector. *Journal of Immunotherapy (Hagerstown, Md.: 1997)* **27**: 339–346.

Hussell, T. & Bell, T. J. (2014) Alveolar macrophages: plasticity in a tissue-specific context. *Nature Reviews Immunology* **14**: 81.

Jin, H., Park, Y., Elly, C. & Liu, Y.-C. (2013) Itch expression by Treg cells controls Th2 inflammatory responses. *The Journal of Clinical Investigation* **123**: 4923–4934.

Johanns, T. M., Ertelt, J. M., Rowe, J. H. & Way, S. S. (2010) Regulatory T cell suppressive potency dictates the balance between bacterial proliferation and clearance during persistent Salmonella infection. *PLoS pathogens* **6**: e1001043.

Jung, Y.-J., LaCourse, R., Ryan, L. & North, R. J. (2002) Evidence inconsistent with a negative influence of T helper 2 cells on protection afforded by a dominant T helper 1 response against Mycobacterium tuberculosis lung infection in mice. *Infection and Immunity* **70**: 6436–6443.

Kaforou, M., Wright, V. J., Oni, T., French, N., Anderson, S. T., Bangani, N., Banwell, C. M., Brent, A. J., Crampin, A. C., Dockrell, H. M., Eley, B., Heyderman, R. S., Hibberd, M. L., Kern, F., Langford, P. R., Ling, L., Mendelson, M., Ottenhoff, T. H., Zgambo, F., Wilkinson, R. J., Coin, L. J. & Levin, M. (2013) Detection of tuberculosis in HIV-infected and -uninfected African adults using whole blood RNA expression signatures: a case-control study. *PLoS medicine* **10**: e1001538.

Kägi, D., Ledermann, B., Bürki, K., Hengartner, H. & Zinkernagel, R. M. (1994) CD8+ T cell-mediated protection against an intracellular bacterium by perforin-dependent cytotoxicity. *European Journal of Immunology* **24**: 3068–3072.

Kaufmann, S. H. E. (1993) Immunity to Intracellular Bacteria. *Annual Review of Immunology* **11**: 129–163.

Kaufmann, S. H. E. (2002) Protection against tuberculosis: cytokines, T cells, and macrophages. *Annals of the Rheumatic Diseases* **61**: ii54.

Keane, J., Gershon, S., Wise, R. P., Mirabile-Levens, E., Kasznica, J., Schwieterman, W. D., Siegel, J. N. & Braun, M. M. (2001) Tuberculosis associated with infliximab, a tumor necrosis factor alpha-neutralizing agent. *The New England Journal of Medicine* **345**: 1098–1104.

Koch, M. A., Tucker-Heard, G., Perdue, N. R., Killebrew, J. R., Urdahl, K. B. & Campbell, D. J. (2009) The transcription factor T-bet controls regulatory T cell homeostasis and function during type 1 inflammation. *Nature Immunology* **10**: 595.

Kocks, C., Marchand, J. B., Gouin, E., d'Hauteville, H., Sansonetti, P. J., Carlier, M. F. & Cossart, P. (1995) The unrelated surface proteins ActA of Listeria monocytogenes and IcsA of Shigella flexneri are sufficient to confer actin-based motility on Listeria innocua and Escherichia coli respectively. *Molecular Microbiology* **18**: 413–423.

Kohm, A. P., McMahon, J. S., Podojil, J. R., Begolka, W. S., DeGutes, M., Kasprowicz, D. J., Ziegler, S. F. & Miller, S. D. (2006) Cutting Edge: Anti-CD25 Monoclonal Antibody Injection Results in the Functional Inactivation, Not Depletion, of CD4$^+$CD25$^+$ T Regulatory Cells. *The Journal of Immunology* **176**: 3301.

Komatsu, N., Mariotti-Ferrandiz, M. E., Wang, Y., Malissen, B., Waldmann, H. & Hori, S. (2009) Heterogeneity of natural Foxp3+ T cells: a committed regulatory T-cell lineage and an uncommitted minor population retaining plasticity. *Proceedings of the National Academy of Sciences of the United States of America* **106**: 1903–1908.

Kursar, M., Koch, M., Mittrücker, H.-W., Nouailles, G., Bonhagen, K., Kamradt, T. & Kaufmann, S. H. E. (2007) Cutting Edge: Regulatory T cells prevent efficient clearance of Mycobacterium tuberculosis. *Journal of Immunology (Baltimore, Md.: 1950)* **178**: 2661–2665.

Kwiatkowska, K. & Sobota, A. (1999) Signaling pathways in phagocytosis. *BioEssays: News and Reviews in Molecular, Cellular and Developmental Biology* **21**: 422–431.

La Cava, A. (2008) Tregs Are Regulated by Cytokines: Implications for Autoimmunity. *Autoimmunity reviews* **8**: 83–87.

Laidlaw, B. J., Cui, W., Amezquita, R. A., Gray, S. M., Guan, T., Lu, Y., Kobayashi, Y., Flavell, R. A., Kleinstein, S. H., Craft, J. & Kaech, S. M. (2015) Production of IL-10 by CD4+ regulatory T cells during the resolution of infection promotes the maturation of memory CD8+ T cells. *Nature immunology* **16**: 871–879.

Lanteri, M. C., O'Brien, K. M., Purtha, W. E., Cameron, M. J., Lund, J. M., Owen, R. E., Heitman, J. W., Custer, B., Hirschkorn, D. F., Tobler, L. H., Kiely, N., Prince, H. E., Ndhlovu, L. C., Nixon, D. F., Kamel, H. T., Kelvin, D. J., Busch, M. P., Rudensky, A. Y., Diamond, M. S. & Norris, P. J. (2009) Tregs control the development of symptomatic West Nile virus infection in humans and mice. *The Journal of Clinical Investigation* **119**: 3266–3277.

Lara-Tejero, M. & Pamer, E. G. (2004) T cell responses to Listeria monocytogenes. *Current Opinion in Microbiology* **7**: 45–50.

Larson, R. P., Shafiani, S. & Urdahl, K. B. (2013) Foxp3(+) regulatory T cells in tuberculosis. *Advances in Experimental Medicine and Biology* **783**: 165–180.

Lee, Y. K., Turner, H., Maynard, C. L., Oliver, J. R., Chen, D., Elson, C. O. & Weaver, C. T. (2009*a*) Late developmental plasticity in the T helper 17 lineage. *Immunity* **30**: 92–107.

Lee, Y. K., Mukasa, R., Hatton, R. D. & Weaver, C. T. (2009*b*) Developmental plasticity of Th17 and Treg cells. *Current Opinion in Immunology* **21**: 274–280.

Leenen, P. J., Canono, B. P., Drevets, D. A., Voerman, J. S. & Campbell, P. A. (1994) TNF-alpha and IFN-gamma stimulate a macrophage precursor cell line to kill Listeria monocytogenes in a nitric oxide-independent manner. *The Journal of Immunology* **153**: 5141.

Leeto, M., Herbert, D. R., Marillier, R., Schwegmann, A., Fick, L. & Brombacher, F. (2006) TH1-dominant granulomatous pathology does not inhibit fibrosis or cause lethality during murine schistosomiasis. *The American Journal of Pathology* **169**: 1701–1712.

Liao, W., Lin, J.-X. & Leonard, W. J. (2011) IL-2 family cytokines: new insights into the complex roles of IL-2 as a broad regulator of T helper cell differentiation. *Current Opinion in Immunology* **23**: 598–604.

Lienhardt, C., Azzurri, A., Amedei, A., Fielding, K., Sillah, J., Sow, O. Y., Bah, B., Benagiano, M., Diallo, A., Manetti, R., Manneh, K., Gustafson, P., Bennett, S., D'Elios, M. M., McAdam, K. & Del Prete, G. (2002) Active tuberculosis in Africa is associated with reduced Th1 and increased Th2 activity in vivo. *European Journal of Immunology* **32**: 1605–1613.

Linnan, M. J., Mascola, L., Lou, X. D., Goulet, V., May, S., Salminen, C., Hird, D. W., Yonekura, M. L., Hayes, P. & Weaver, R. (1988) Epidemic listeriosis associated with Mexican-style cheese. *The New England Journal of Medicine* **319**: 823–828.

Lochner, M., Kastenmüller, K., Neuenhahn, M., Weighardt, H., Busch, D. H., Reindl, W. & Förster, I. (2008) Decreased Susceptibility of Mice to Infection with <em>Listeria monocytogenes</em> in the Absence of Interleukin-18. *Infection and Immunity* **76**: 3881.

Locksley, R. M. (1993) Interleukin 12 in host defense against microbial pathogens. *Proceedings of the National Academy of Sciences of the United States of America* **90**: 5879–5880.

Lücke, K., Yan, I., Krohn, S., Volmari, A., Klinge, S., Schmid, J., Schumacher, V., Steinmetz, O. M., Rose-John, S. & Mittrücker, H.-W. (2018) Control of Listeria monocytogenes infection requires classical IL-6 signaling in myeloid cells. *PLOS ONE* **13**: e0203395.

Lund, J. M., Hsing, L., Pham, T. T. & Rudensky, A. Y. (2008) Coordination of Early Protective Immunity to Viral Infection by Regulatory T Cells. *Science (New York, N.Y.)* **320**: 1220–1224.

Ma, B., He, F., Jablonska, J., Winkelbach, S., Lindenmaier, W., Zeng, A.-P. & Dittmar, K. E. J. (2007) Six-color segmentation of multicolor images in the infection studies of Listeria monocytogenes. *Microscopy Research and Technique* **70**: 171–178.

MacMicking, J. D., Taylor, G. A. & McKinney, J. D. (2003) Immune control of tuberculosis by IFN-gamma-inducible LRG-47. *Science (New York, N.Y.)* **302**: 654–659.

Maerten, P., Shen, C., Bullens, D. M. A., Van Assche, G., Van Gool, S., Geboes, K., Rutgeerts, P. & Ceuppens, J. L. (2005) Effects of interleukin 4 on CD25+CD4+ regulatory T cell function. *Journal of Autoimmunity* **25**: 112–120.

Maertzdorf, J., Repsilber, D., Parida, S. K., Stanley, K., Roberts, T., Black, G., Walzl, G. & Kaufmann, S. H. E. (2011) Human gene expression profiles of susceptibility and resistance in tuberculosis. *Genes and Immunity* **12**: 15–22.

Mahomed, H., Hawkridge, T., Verver, S., Geiter, L., Hatherill, M., Abrahams, D.-A., Ehrlich, R., Hanekom, W. A., Hussey, G. D. & SATVI Adolescent Study Team (2011) Predictive factors for latent tuberculosis infection among adolescents in a high-burden area in South Africa. *The International Journal of Tuberculosis and Lung Disease: The Official Journal of the International Union Against Tuberculosis and Lung Disease* **15**: 331–336.

Marillier, R. G., Brombacher, T. M., Dewals, B., Leeto, M., Barkhuizen, M., Govender, D., Kellaway, L., Horsnell, W. G. C. & Brombacher, F. (2010) IL-4R{alpha}-responsive smooth muscle cells increase intestinal hypercontractility and contribute to resistance during acute Schistosomiasis. *American Journal of Physiology. Gastrointestinal and Liver Physiology* **298**: G943-951.

Marin, N. D., París, S. C., Vélez, V. M., Rojas, C. A., Rojas, M. & García, L. F. (2010) Regulatory T cell frequency and modulation of IFN-gamma and IL-17 in active and latent tuberculosis. *Tuberculosis (Edinburgh, Scotland)* **90**: 252–261.

Martinez, F. O., Helming, L. & Gordon, S. (2009) Alternative activation of macrophages: an immunologic functional perspective. *Annual Review of Immunology* **27**: 451–483.

Massoud, A. H., Charbonnier, L.-M., Lopez, D., Pellegrini, M., Phipatanakul, W. & Chatila, T. A. (2016) An asthma-associated IL4R variant exacerbates airway inflammation by promoting conversion of regulatory T cells to TH17-like cells. *Nature Medicine* **22**: 1013.

McIlwain, D. R., Lang, P. A., Maretzky, T., Hamada, K., Ohishi, K., Maney, S. K., Berger, T., Murthy, A., Duncan, G., Xu, H. C., Lang, K. S., Häussinger, D., Wakeham, A., Itie-Youten, A., Khokha, R., Ohashi, P. S., Blobel, C. P. & Mak, T. W. (2012) iRhom2 Regulation of TACE Controls TNF-Mediated Protection Against Listeria and Responses to LPS. *Science* **335**: 229.

Medzhitov, R. & Janeway, C. (2000) Innate Immunity. *New England Journal of Medicine* **343**: 338–344.

Mercado, R., Vijh, S., Allen, S. E., Kerksiek, K., Pilip, I. M. & Pamer, E. G. (2000) Early Programming of T Cell Populations Responding to Bacterial Infection. *The Journal of Immunology* **165**: 6833.

Messingham, K. A. N., Badovinac, V. P., Jabbari, A. & Harty, J. T. (2007) A role for IFN-gamma from antigen-specific CD8+ T cells in protective immunity to Listeria monocytogenes. *Journal of Immunology (Baltimore, Md.: 1950)* **179**: 2457–2466.

Miettinen, M. K., Siitonen, A., Heiskanen, P., Haajanen, H., Björkroth, K. J. & Korkeala, H. J. (1999) Molecular Epidemiology of an Outbreak of Febrile Gastroenteritis Caused by Listeria monocytogenes in Cold-Smoked Rainbow Trout. *Journal of Clinical Microbiology* **37**: 2358–2360.

Mihret, A., Bekele, Y., Loxton, A. G., Aseffa, A., Howe, R. & Walzl, G. (2012) Plasma Level of IL-4 Differs in Patients Infected with Different Modern Lineages of M. tuberculosis. *Journal of Tropical Medicine*.

Mihret, A., Bekele, Y., Bobosha, K., Kidd, M., Aseffa, A., Howe, R. & Walzl, G. (2013) Plasma cytokines and chemokines differentiate between active disease and non-active tuberculosis infection. *The Journal of Infection* **66**: 357–365.

Mitra, S. & Leonard, W. J. (2018) Biology of IL-2 and its therapeutic modulation: Mechanisms and strategies. *Journal of Leukocyte Biology* **103**: 643–655.

Mogues, T., Goodrich, M. E., Ryan, L., LaCourse, R. & North, R. J. (2001) The Relative Importance of T Cell Subsets in Immunity and Immunopathology of Airborne

Mycobacterium tuberculosis Infection in Mice. *The Journal of Experimental Medicine* **193**: 271–280.

Morse, D., Brothwell, D. R. & Ucko, P. J. (1964) TUBERCULOSIS IN ANCIENT EGYPT. *The American Review of Respiratory Disease* **90**: 524–541.

Mosser, D. M. & Edwards, J. P. (2008) Exploring the full spectrum of macrophage activation. *Nature Reviews Immunology* **8**: 958.

Mouchacca, P., Schmitt-Verhulst, A.-M. & Boyer, C. (2013) Visualization of cytolytic T cell differentiation and granule exocytosis with T cells from mice expressing active fluorescent granzyme B. *PloS One* **8**: e67239.

Mouchacca, P., Chasson, L., Frick, M., Foray, C., Schmitt-Verhulst, A.-M. & Boyer, C. (2015) Visualization of granzyme B-expressing CD8 T cells during primary and secondary immune responses to Listeria monocytogenes. *Immunology* **145**: 24–33.

Murphy, K. (2011) *Janeway's Immunobiology*. Garland Science.

Murray, E. G. D., Webb, R. A. & Swann, M. B. R. (1926) A disease of rabbits characterised by a large mononuclear leucocytosis, caused by a hitherto undescribed bacillus Bacterium monocytogenes (n.sp.). *The Journal of Pathology and Bacteriology* **29**: 407–439.

Murray, P. J. & Wynn, T. A. (2011) Protective and pathogenic functions of macrophage subsets. *Nature Reviews Immunology* **11**: 723–737.

Murray, P. J. & Young, R. A. (1999) Increased Antimycobacterial Immunity in Interleukin-10-Deficient Mice. *Infection and Immunity* **67**: 3087–3095.

Ndlovu, H. & Marakalala, M. J. (2016) Granulomas and Inflammation: Host-Directed Therapies for Tuberculosis. *Frontiers in Immunology* **7**: 434.

Ngai, P., McCormick, S., Small, C., Zhang, X., Zganiacz, A., Aoki, N. & Xing, Z. (2007) Gamma Interferon Responses of CD4 and CD8 T-Cell Subsets Are Quantitatively Different and Independent of Each Other during Pulmonary Mycobacterium bovis BCG Infection. *Infection and Immunity* **75**: 2244–2252.

Noben-Trauth, N., Paul, W. E. & Sacks, D. L. (1999) IL-4- and IL-4 receptor-deficient BALB/c mice reveal differences in susceptibility to Leishmania major parasite substrains. *Journal of Immunology (Baltimore, Md.: 1950)* **162**: 6132–6140.

North, R. J. (1998) Mice incapable of making IL-4 or IL-10 display normal resistance to infection with Mycobacterium tuberculosis. *Clinical and Experimental Immunology* **113**: 55–58.

Noval Rivas, M., Burton, O. T., Wise, P., Charbonnier, L.-M., Georgiev, P., Oettgen, H. C., Rachid, R. & Chatila, T. A. (2015) Regulatory T Cell Reprogramming toward a Th2-Cell-like Lineage Impairs Oral Tolerance and Promotes Food Allergy. *Immunity* **42**: 512–523.

Nunes-Alves, C., Booty, M. G., Carpenter, S. M., Jayaraman, P., Rothchild, A. C. & Behar, S. M. (2014) In search of a new paradigm for protective immunity to TB. *Nature reviews. Microbiology* **12**: 289–299.

O'Garra, A., Redford, P. S., McNab, F. W., Bloom, C. I., Wilkinson, R. J. & Berry, M. P. R. (2013) The Immune Response in Tuberculosis. *Annual Review of Immunology* **31**: 475–527.

Omenetti, S. & Pizarro, T. T. (2015) The Treg/Th17 Axis: A Dynamic Balance Regulated by the Gut Microbiome. *Frontiers in Immunology* **6**.

Ordway, D. J., Martins, M. S., Costa, L. M., Freire, M. S., Arroz, M. J., Dockrell, H. M. & Ventura, F. A. (2005) [Increased IL-4 production in response to virulent Mycobacterium tuberculosis in tuberculosis patients with advanced disease]. *Acta Medica Portuguesa* **18**: 27–36.

O'Shea, J. J. & Paul, W. E. (2010) Mechanisms Underlying Lineage Commitment and Plasticity of Helper CD4$^+$ T Cells. *Science* **327**: 1098.

Pace, L., Pioli, C. & Doria, G. (2005) IL-4 Modulation of CD4+CD25+ T Regulatory Cell-Mediated Suppression. *The Journal of Immunology* **174**: 7645–7653.

Pai, M., Behr, M. A., Dowdy, D., Dheda, K., Divangahi, M., Boehme, C. C., Ginsberg, A., Swaminathan, S., Spigelman, M., Getahun, H., Menzies, D. & Raviglione, M. (2016) Tuberculosis. *Nature Reviews Disease Primers* **2**: 16076.

Pamer, E. G. (2004) Immune responses to Listeria monocytogenes. *Nature Reviews Immunology* **4**: 812–823.

Pandiyan, P., Conti, H. R., Zheng, L., Peterson, A. C., Mathern, D. R., Hernández-Santos, N., Edgerton, M., Gaffen, S. L. & Lenardo, M. J. (2011) CD4+ CD25+ Foxp3+ regulatory T cells promote Th17 cells in vitro and enhance host resistance in mouse Candida albicans Th17 cell infection model. *Immunity* **34**: 422–434.

Parida, S. K., Poiret, T., Zhenjiang, L., Meng, Q., Heyckendorf, J., Lange, C., Ambati, A. S., Rao, M. V., Valentini, D., Ferrara, G., Rangelova, E., Dodoo, E., Zumla, A. & Maeurer, M. (2015) T-Cell Therapy: Options for Infectious Diseases. *Clinical Infectious Diseases: An Official Publication of the Infectious Diseases Society of America* **61**: S217–S224.

Pelly, V. S., Coomes, S. M., Kannan, Y., Gialitakis, M., Entwistle, L. J., Perez-Lloret, J., Czieso, S., Okoye, I. S., Rückerl, D., Allen, J. E., Brombacher, F. & Wilson, M. S. (2017) Interleukin 4 promotes the development of ex-Foxp3 Th2 cells during immunity to intestinal helminths. *The Journal of Experimental Medicine* **214**: 1809–1826.

Pirie, J. H. H. (1940) Listeria: Change of Name for a Genus Bacteria. *Nature* **145**: 264.

Pizarro-Cerdá, J. & Cossart, P. (2006) Subversion of cellular functions by Listeria monocytogenes. *The Journal of Pathology* **208**: 215–223.

Pope, C., Kim, S. K., Marzo, A., Masopust, D., Williams, K., Jiang, J., Shen, H. & Lefrançois, L. (2001) Organ-specific regulation of the CD8 T cell response to Listeria monocytogenes infection. *Journal of Immunology (Baltimore, Md.: 1950)* **166**: 3402–3409.

Potian, J. A., Rafi, W., Bhatt, K., McBride, A., Gause, W. C. & Salgame, P. (2011) Preexisting helminth infection induces inhibition of innate pulmonary anti-tuberculosis defense by engaging the IL-4 receptor pathway. *The Journal of Experimental Medicine* **208**: 1863–1874.

Prochazkova, J., Fric, J., Pokorna, K., Neuwirth, A., Krulova, M., Zajicova, A. & Holan, V. (2009) Distinct regulatory roles of transforming growth factor-β and interleukin-4 in the development and maintenance of natural and induced CD4+ CD25+ Foxp3+ regulatory T cells. *Immunology* **128**: e670–e678.

Quinn, K. M., McHugh, R. S., Rich, F. J., Goldsack, L. M., de Lisle, G. W., Buddle, B. M., Delahunt, B. & Kirman, J. R. (2006) Inactivation of CD4+ CD25+ regulatory T cells during early mycobacterial infection increases cytokine production but does not affect pathogen load. *Immunology and Cell Biology* **84**: 467–474.

Radwanska, M., Cutler, A. J., Hoving, J. C., Magez, S., Holscher, C., Bohms, A., Arendse, B., Kirsch, R., Hunig, T., Alexander, J., Kaye, P. & Brombacher, F. (2007) Deletion of IL-4Rα on CD4 T Cells Renders BALB/c Mice Resistant to Leishmania major Infection. *PLOS Pathogens* **3**: e68.

Reiley, W. W., Calayag, M. D., Wittmer, S. T., Huntington, J. L., Pearl, J. E., Fountain, J. J., Martino, C. A., Roberts, A. D., Cooper, A. M., Winslow, G. M. & Woodland, D. L. (2008) ESAT-6-specific CD4 T cell responses to aerosol Mycobacterium tuberculosis infection are initiated in the mediastinal lymph nodes. *Proceedings of the National Academy of Sciences of the United States of America* **105**: 10961–10966.

Rogers, H. W. & Unanue, E. R. (1993) Neutrophils are involved in acute, nonspecific resistance to Listeria monocytogenes in mice. *Infection and Immunity* **61**: 5090.

Romagnoli, P. A., Fu, H. H., Qiu, Z., Khairallah, C., Pham, Q. M., Puddington, L., Khanna, K. M., Lefrançois, L. & Sheridan, B. S. (2017) Differentiation of distinct long-lived memory CD4 T cells in intestinal tissues after oral Listeria monocytogenes infection. *Mucosal Immunology* **10**: 520–530.

Rook, G. A. W. (2007) Th2 cytokines in susceptibility to tuberculosis. *Current Molecular Medicine* **7**: 327–337.

Rook, G. A. W., Hernandez-Pando, R., Dheda, K. & Teng Seah, G. (2004) IL-4 in tuberculosis: implications for vaccine design. *Trends in Immunology* **25**: 483–488.

Rowe, J. H., Ertelt, J. M., Aguilera, M. N., Farrar, M. A. & Way, S. S. (2011) Foxp3(+) regulatory T cell expansion required for sustaining pregnancy compromises host defense against prenatal bacterial pathogens. *Cell Host & Microbe* **10**: 54–64.

Rowe, J. H., Ertelt, J. M. & Way, S. S. (2012) Foxp3+ regulatory T cells, immune stimulation and host defence against infection. *Immunology* **136**: 1–10.

Roy, E., Brennan, J., Jolles, S. & Lowrie, D. B. (2008) Beneficial effect of anti-interleukin-4 antibody when administered in a murine model of tuberculosis infection. *Tuberculosis* **88**: 197–202.

Sahibzada, H. A., Khurshid, Z., Khan, R. S., Naseem, M., Siddique, K. M., Mali, M. & Zafar, M. S. (2017) Salivary IL-8, IL-6 and TNF-α as Potential Diagnostic Biomarkers for Oral Cancer. *Diagnostics (Basel, Switzerland)* **7**.

Sanjabi, S., Zenewicz, L. A., Kamanaka, M. & Flavell, R. A. (2009) Anti-inflammatory and pro-inflammatory roles of TGF-beta, IL-10, and IL-22 in immunity and autoimmunity. *Current opinion in pharmacology* **9**: 447–453.

Saraiva, M., Christensen, J. R., Veldhoen, M., Murphy, T. L., Murphy, K. M. & O'Garra, A. (2009) Interleukin-10 production by Th1 cells requires interleukin-12-induced STAT4 transcription factor and ERK MAP kinase activation by high antigen dose. *Immunity* **31**: 209–219.

Sawant, D. V. & Vignali, D. A. A. (2014) Once a Treg, always a Treg? *Immunological reviews* **259**: 173–191.

Sawant, D. V., Sehra, S., Nguyen, E. T., Jadhav, R., Englert, K., Shinnakasu, R., Hangoc, G., Broxmeyer, H. E., Nakayama, T., Perumal, N. B., Kaplan, M. H. & Dent, A. L. (2012) Bcl6 controls the Th2 inflammatory activity of regulatory T cells by repressing Gata3 function. *Journal of Immunology (Baltimore, Md.: 1950)* **189**: 4759–4769.

Schauf, V., Rom, W. N., Smith, K. A., Sampaio, E. P., Meyn, P. A., Tramontana, J. M., Cohn, Z. A. & Kaplan, G. (1993) Cytokine Gene Activation and Modified Responsiveness to Interleukin-2 in the Blood of Tuberculosis Patients. *The Journal of Infectious Diseases* **168**: 1056–1059.

Schlech, W. F., Lavigne, P. M., Bortolussi, R. A., Allen, A. C., Haldane, E. V., Wort, A. J., Hightower, A. W., Johnson, S. E., King, S. H., Nicholls, E. S. & Broome, C. V. (1983) Epidemic listeriosis--evidence for transmission by food. *The New England Journal of Medicine* **308**: 203–206.

Scott, P. (1993) IL-12: initiation cytokine for cell-mediated immunity. *Science* **260**: 496.

Scott-Browne, J. P., Shafiani, S., Tucker-Heard, G., Ishida-Tsubota, K., Fontenot, J. D., Rudensky, A. Y., Bevan, M. J. & Urdahl, K. B. (2007) Expansion and function of Foxp3-expressing T regulatory cells during tuberculosis. *The Journal of Experimental Medicine* **204**: 2159–2169.

Seah, G. T., Scott, G. M. & Rook, G. A. (2000) Type 2 cytokine gene activation and its relationship to extent of disease in patients with tuberculosis. *The Journal of Infectious Diseases* **181**: 385–389.

Seder, R. A. & Paul, W. E. (1994) Acquisition of Lymphokine-Producing Phenotype by CD4+ T Cells. *Annual Review of Immunology* **12**: 635–673.

Seki, E., Tsutsui, H., Tsuji, N. M., Hayashi, N., Adachi, K., Nakano, H., Futatsugi-Yumikura, S., Takeuchi, O., Hoshino, K., Akira, S., Fujimoto, J. & Nakanishi, K. (2002) Critical roles of myeloid differentiation factor 88-dependent proinflammatory cytokine release in early phase clearance of Listeria monocytogenes in mice. *Journal of Immunology (Baltimore, Md.: 1950)* **169**: 3863–3868.

Setoguchi, R., Hori, S., Takahashi, T. & Sakaguchi, S. (2005) Homeostatic maintenance of natural Foxp3(+) CD25(+) CD4(+) regulatory T cells by interleukin (IL)-2 and induction of autoimmune disease by IL-2 neutralization. *The Journal of experimental medicine* **201**: 723–735.

Shafiani, S., Tucker-Heard, G., Kariyone, A., Takatsu, K. & Urdahl, K. B. (2010) Pathogen-specific regulatory T cells delay the arrival of effector T cells in the lung during early tuberculosis. *The Journal of Experimental Medicine* **207**: 1409–1420.

Shedlock, D. J., Whitmire, J. K., Tan, J., MacDonald, A. S., Ahmed, R. & Shen, H. (2003) Role of CD4 T cell help and costimulation in CD8 T cell responses during Listeria monocytogenes infection. *Journal of Immunology (Baltimore, Md.: 1950)* **170**: 2053–2063.

Shen, H., Miller, J. F., Fan, X., Kolwyck, D., Ahmed, R. & Harty, J. T. (1998) Compartmentalization of Bacterial Antigens: Differential Effects on Priming of CD8 T Cells and Protective Immunity. *Cell* **92**: 535–545.

Shen, Y., Naujokas, M., Park, M. & Ireton, K. (2000) InIB-dependent internalization of Listeria is mediated by the Met receptor tyrosine kinase. *Cell* **103**: 501–510.

Shi, C., Hohl, T. M., Leiner, I., Equinda, M. J., Fan, X. & Pamer, E. G. (2011) Ly6G+ neutrophils are dispensable for defense against systemic Listeria monocytogenes infection. *Journal of Immunology (Baltimore, Md.: 1950)* **187**: 5293–5298.

Silver, N., Cotroneo, E., Proctor, G., Osailan, S., Paterson, K. L. & Carpenter, G. H. (2008) Selection of housekeeping genes for gene expression studies in the adult rat submandibular gland under normal, inflamed, atrophic and regenerative states. *BMC molecular biology* **9**: 64.

Smigiel, K. S., Srivastava, S., Stolley, J. M. & Campbell, D. J. (2014) Regulatory T cell homeostasis: steady-state maintenance and modulation during inflammation. *Immunological reviews* **259**: 40–59.

Smith, G. A., Portnoy, D. A. & Theriot, J. A. (1995) Asymmetric distribution of the Listeria monocytogenes ActA protein is required and sufficient to direct actin-based motility. *Molecular Microbiology* **17**: 945–951.

Smith, S. M., Klein, M. R., Malin, A. S., Sillah, J., McAdam, K. P. W. J. & Dockrell, H. M. (2002) Decreased IFN- gamma and increased IL-4 production by human CD8(+) T cells in response to Mycobacterium tuberculosis in tuberculosis patients. *Tuberculosis (Edinburgh, Scotland)* **82**: 7–13.

Sousa, A. O., Mazzaccaro, R. J., Russell, R. G., Lee, F. K., Turner, O. C., Hong, S., Van Kaer, L. & Bloom, B. R. (2000) Relative contributions of distinct MHC class I-dependent cell populations in protection to tuberculosis infection in mice. *Proceedings of the National Academy of Sciences of the United States of America* **97**: 4204–4208.

Sousa, S., Cabanes, D., Bougnères, L., Lecuit, M., Sansonetti, P., Tran-Van-Nhieu, G. & Cossart, P. (2007) Src, cortactin and Arp2/3 complex are required for E-cadherin-mediated internalization of Listeria into cells. *Cellular Microbiology* **9**: 2629–2643.

de Souza Santos, M. & Orth, K. (2015) Subversion of the cytoskeleton by intracellular bacteria: lessons from Listeria, Salmonella, and Vibrio. *Cellular microbiology* **17**: 164–173.

Spaner, D., Raju, K., Rabinovich, B. & Miller, R. G. (1999) A Role for Perforin in Activation-Induced T Cell Death In Vivo: Increased Expansion of Allogeneic Perforin-Deficient T Cells in SCID mice. *The Journal of Immunology* **162**: 1192–1199.

Stachowiak, R., Lyzniak, M., Budziszewska, B. K., Roeske, K., Bielecki, J., Hoser, G. & Kawiak, J. (2012) Cytotoxicity of bacterial metabolic products, including listeriolysin O, on leukocyte targets. *Journal of Biomedicine & Biotechnology* **2012**: 954375.

Sun, J. C. & Bevan, M. J. (2003) Defective CD8 T Cell Memory Following Acute Infection Without CD4 T Cell Help. *Science* **300**: 339.

Suvas, S., Kumaraguru, U., Pack, C. D., Lee, S. & Rouse, B. T. (2003) CD4+CD25+ T Cells Regulate Virus-specific Primary and Memory CD8+ T Cell Responses. *The Journal of Experimental Medicine* **198**: 889–901.

Szabo, S. J., Kim, S. T., Costa, G. L., Zhang, X., Fathman, C. G. & Glimcher, L. H. (2000) A Novel Transcription Factor, T-bet, Directs Th1 Lineage Commitment. *Cell* **100**: 655–669.

Szalay, G., Ladel, C. H., Blum, C. & Kaufmann, S. H. (1996) IL-4 neutralization or TNF-alpha treatment ameliorate disease by an intracellular pathogen in IFN-gamma receptor-deficient mice. *The Journal of Immunology* **157**: 4746–4750.

Takeuchi, A. & Saito, T. (2017) CD4 CTL, a Cytotoxic Subset of CD4+ T Cells, Their Differentiation and Function. *Frontiers in Immunology* **8**.

Talwar, A., Arun, K. V., Kumar, T. S. S. & Clements, J. (2013) Plasticity of T helper cell subsets: Implications in periodontal disease. *Journal of Indian Society of Periodontology* **17**: 288–291.

Th2 cells: help for helminths (1994) *The Journal of Experimental Medicine* **179**: 1405–1407.

Thäle, C. & Kiderlen, A. F. (2005) Sources of interferon-gamma (IFN-γ) in early immune response to Listeria monocytogenes. *Immunobiology* **210**: 673–683.

Thieu, V. T., Yu, Q., Chang, H.-C., Yeh, N., Nguyen, E. T., Sehra, S. & Kaplan, M. H. (2008) Stat4 is required for T-bet to promote IL-12-dependent Th1 fate determination. *Immunity* **29**: 679–690.

Thompson, E. G., Du, Y., Malherbe, S. T., Shankar, S., Braun, J., Valvo, J., Ronacher, K., Tromp, G., Tabb, D. L., Alland, D., Shenai, S., Via, L. E., Warwick, J., Aderem, A., Scriba, T. J., Winter, J., Walzl, G., Zak, D. E. & Catalysis TB–Biomarker Consortium (2017) Host blood RNA signatures predict the outcome of tuberculosis treatment. *Tuberculosis (Edinburgh, Scotland)* **107**: 48–58.

Torrado, E. & Cooper, A. M. (2010) IL-17 and Th17 cells in tuberculosis. *Cytokine & growth factor reviews* **21**: 455–462.

Tu, L., Chen, J., Zhang, H. & Duan, L. (2017) Interleukin-4 Inhibits Regulatory T Cell Differentiation through Regulating CD103+ Dendritic Cells. *Frontiers in Immunology* **8**.

Tvinnereim, A. R., Hamilton, S. E. & Harty, J. T. (2002*a*) CD8$^+$-T-Cell Response to Secreted and Nonsecreted Antigens Delivered by Recombinant <em>Listeria monocytogenes</em> during Secondary Infection. *Infection and Immunity* **70**: 153.

Tvinnereim, A. R., Hamilton, S. E. & Harty, J. T. (2002*b*) CD8+-T-Cell Response to Secreted and Nonsecreted Antigens Delivered by Recombinant Listeria monocytogenes during Secondary Infection. *Infection and Immunity* **70**: 153–162.

Ulges, A., Klein, M., Reuter, S., Gerlitzki, B., Hoffmann, M., Grebe, N., Staudt, V., Stergiou, N., Bohn, T., Brühl, T.-J., Muth, S., Yurugi, H., Rajalingam, K., Bellinghausen, I., Tuettenberg, A., Hahn, S., Reißig, S., Haben, I., Zipp, F., Waisman, A., Probst, H.-C., Beilhack, A., Buchou, T., Filhol-Cochet, O., Boldyreff, B., Breloer, M., Jonuleit, H., Schild, H., Schmitt, E. & Bopp, T. (2015) Protein kinase CK2 enables regulatory T cells to suppress excessive TH2 responses in vivo. *Nature Immunology* **16**: 267–275.

Unanue, E. R. (1997) Studies in listeriosis show the strong symbiosis between the innate cellular system and the T-cell response. *Immunological Reviews* **158**: 11–25.

Urdahl, K., Shafiani, S. & Ernst, J. (2011) Initiation and regulation of T-cell responses in tuberculosis. *Mucosal immunology* **4**: 288–293.

Vazquez-Boland, J. A., Kocks, C., Dramsi, S., Ohayon, H., Geoffroy, C., Mengaud, J. & Cossart, P. (1992) Nucleotide sequence of the lecithinase operon of Listeria monocytogenes and possible role of lecithinase in cell-to-cell spread. *Infection and Immunity* **60**: 219–230.

Vázquez-Boland, J. A., Kuhn, M., Berche, P., Chakraborty, T., Domínguez-Bernal, G., Goebel, W., González-Zorn, B., Wehland, J. & Kreft, J. (2001) Listeria Pathogenesis and Molecular Virulence Determinants. *Clinical Microbiology Reviews* **14**: 584–640.

Veldhoen, M., Uyttenhove, C., van Snick, J., Helmby, H., Westendorf, A., Buer, J., Martin, B., Wilhelm, C. & Stockinger, B. (2008) Transforming growth factor-β 'reprograms' the differentiation of T helper 2 cells and promotes an interleukin 9–producing subset. *Nature Immunology* **9**: 1341–1346.

Vieira, O. V., Botelho, R. J. & Grinstein, S. (2002) Phagosome maturation: aging gracefully. *The Biochemical Journal* **366**: 689–704.

Vilček, J. & Feldmann, M. (2004) Historical review: Cytokines as therapeutics and targets of therapeutics. *Trends in Pharmacological Sciences* **25**: 201–209.

Wagner, R. D. & Czuprynski, C. J. (1993) Cytokine mRNA expression in livers of mice infected with Listeria monocytogenes. *Journal of Leukocyte Biology* **53**: 525–531.

Waite, J. C., Leiner, I., Lauer, P., Rae, C. S., Barbet, G., Zheng, H., Portnoy, D. A., Pamer, E. G. & Dustin, M. L. (2011) Dynamic imaging of the effector immune response to listeria infection in vivo. *PLoS pathogens* **7**: e1001326–e1001326.

Wallgren, A. (1948) The time-table of tuberculosis. *Tubercle* **29**: 245–251.

Wang, N., Strugnell, R., Wijburg, O. & Brodnicki, T. (2011) Measuring bacterial load and immune responses in mice infected with Listeria monocytogenes. *Journal of Visualized Experiments: JoVE.*

Wang, T. & Secombes, C. J. (2013) The cytokine networks of adaptive immunity in fish. *Fish & Shellfish Immunology* **35**: 1703–1718.

Wang, Y., Souabni, A., Flavell, R. A. & Wan, Y. Y. (2010) An intrinsic mechanism predisposes Foxp3-expressing regulatory T cells to Th2 conversion in vivo. *Journal of Immunology (Baltimore, Md.: 1950)* **185**: 5983–5992.

Wei, G., Wei, L., Zhu, J., Zang, C., Hu-Li, J., Yao, Z., Cui, K., Kanno, Y., Roh, T.-Y., Watford, W. T., Schones, D. E., Peng, W., Sun, H., Paul, W. E., O'Shea, J. J. & Zhao, K. (2009) Global Mapping of H3K4me3 and H3K27me3 Reveals Specificity and Plasticity in Lineage Fate Determination of Differentiating CD4+ T Cells. *Immunity* **30**: 155–167.

Welsh, K. J., Risin, S. A., Actor, J. K. & Hunter, R. L. (2011) Immunopathology of postprimary tuberculosis: increased T-regulatory cells and DEC-205-positive foamy macrophages in cavitary lesions. *Clinical & Developmental Immunology* **2011**: 307631.

WHO (2018) Tuberculosis.

Wills-Karp, M. & Finkelman, F. D. (2008) Untangling the Complex Web of IL-4– and IL-13–Mediated Signaling Pathways. *Science Signaling* **1**: pe55.

Wing, K. & Sakaguchi, S. (2010) Regulatory T cells exert checks and balances on self tolerance and autoimmunity. *Nature Immunology* **11**: 7–13.

Witter, A. R., Okunnu, B. M. & Berg, R. E. (2016) The Essential Role of Neutrophils During Infection with the Intracellular Bacterial Pathogen Listeria monocytogenes. *Journal of immunology (Baltimore, Md. : 1950)* **197**: 1557–1565.

Wolf, A. J., Linas, B., Trevejo-Nuñez, G. J., Kincaid, E., Tamura, T., Takatsu, K. & Ernst, J. D. (2007) Mycobacterium tuberculosis infects dendritic cells with high frequency and impairs their function in vivo. *Journal of Immunology (Baltimore, Md.: 1950)* **179**: 2509–2519.

Wolf, A. J., Desvignes, L., Linas, B., Banaiee, N., Tamura, T., Takatsu, K. & Ernst, J. D. (2008) Initiation of the adaptive immune response to Mycobacterium tuberculosis depends on antigen production in the local lymph node, not the lungs. *The Journal of Experimental Medicine* **205**: 105–115.

Wolf, B. J. & Princiotta, M. F. (2013) Processing of recombinant Listeria monocytogenes proteins for MHC class I presentation follows a dedicated, high-efficiency pathway. *Journal of Immunology (Baltimore, Md.: 1950)* **190**: 2501–2509.

Wong, P. & Pamer, E. G. (2001) Cutting edge: antigen-independent CD8 T cell proliferation. *Journal of Immunology (Baltimore, Md.: 1950)* **166**: 5864–5868.

World Health Organization (WHO) (2018) Listeriosis–South Africa. *Disease outbreak news. http://www. who. int/csr/don/28-march-2018-listeriosis-south-africa/en/. Accessed* **2**.

Xu, L., Kitani, A., Fuss, I. & Strober, W. (2007) Cutting Edge: Regulatory T Cells Induce CD4+CD25−Foxp3− T Cells or Are Self-Induced to Become Th17 Cells in the Absence of Exogenous TGF-β. *The Journal of Immunology* **178**: 6725–6729.

Yin, Y., Lian, K., Zhao, D., Tao, C., Chen, X., Tan, W., Wang, X., Xu, Z., Hu, M., Rao, Y., Zhou, X., Pan, Z., Zhang, X. & Jiao, X. (2017) A Promising Listeria-Vectored Vaccine Induces Th1-Type Immune Responses and Confers Protection Against Tuberculosis. *Frontiers in Cellular and Infection Microbiology* **7**.

Zaiss, D. M. W., Sijts, A. J. A. M. & Mosmann, T. R. (2008) Enumeration of Cytotoxic CD8 T Cells Ex Vivo during the Response to Listeria monocytogenes Infection. *Infection and Immunity* **76**: 4609–4614.

Zelenay, S., Lopes-Carvalho, T., Caramalho, I., Moraes-Fontes, M. F., Rebelo, M. & Demengeot, J. (2005) Foxp3+ CD25- CD4 T cells constitute a reservoir of committed regulatory cells that regain CD25 expression upon homeostatic expansion. *Proceedings of the National Academy of Sciences of the United States of America* **102**: 4091–4096.

Zenewicz, L. A. & Shen, H. (2007a) Innate and adaptive immune responses to Listeria monocytogenes: A short overview. *Microbes and infection / Institut Pasteur* **9**: 1208–1215.

Zenewicz, L. A. & Shen, H. (2007b) Innate and adaptive immune responses to Listeria monocytogenes: a short overview. *Microbes and Infection* **9**: 1208–1215.

Zhai, Y., Franco, L. M., Atmar, R. L., Quarles, J. M., Arden, N., Bucasas, K. L., Wells, J. M., Niño, D., Wang, X., Zapata, G. E., Shaw, C. A., Belmont, J. W. & Couch, R. B. (2015) Host Transcriptional Response to Influenza and Other Acute Respiratory Viral Infections--A Prospective Cohort Study. *PLoS pathogens* **11**: e1004869.

Zhou, X., Bailey-Bucktrout, S. L., Jeker, L. T., Penaranda, C., Martínez-Llordella, M., Ashby, M., Nakayama, M., Rosenthal, W. & Bluestone, J. A. (2009) Instability of the transcription factor Foxp3 leads to the generation of pathogenic memory T cells in vivo. *Nature Immunology* **10**: 1000–1007.

Zhu, J. (2010) Transcriptional regulation of Th2 cell differentiation. *Immunology and Cell Biology* **88**: 244–249.

Zhu, W., Hu, Z., Liao, X., Chen, X., Huang, W., Zhong, Y. & Zeng, Z. (2017) A new mutation site in the AIRE gene causes autoimmune polyendocrine syndrome type 1. *Immunogenetics* **69**: 643–651.

Zimmerer, J. M., Horne, P. H., Fisher, M. G., Pham, T. A., Lunsford, K. E., Ringwald, B. A., Avila, C. L. & Bumgardner, G. L. (2016) Unique CD8+ T cell Mediated Immune Responses Primed in the Liver. *Transplantation* **100**: 1907–1915.

Zimmerman, M. R. (1979) Pulmonary and osseous tuberculosis in an Egyptian mummy. *Bulletin of the New York Academy of Medicine* **55**: 604–608.

APPENDIX

Lymphoid gating

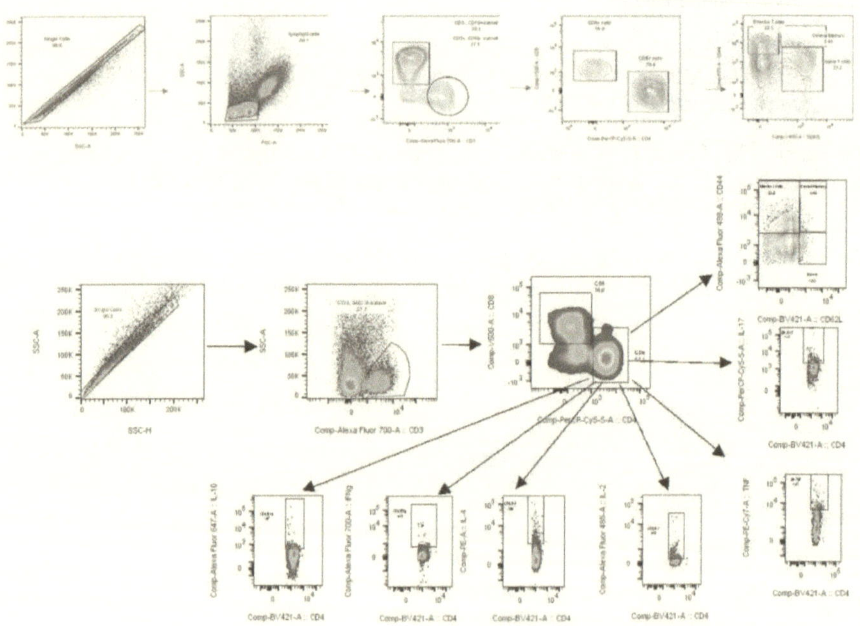

Myeloid gating

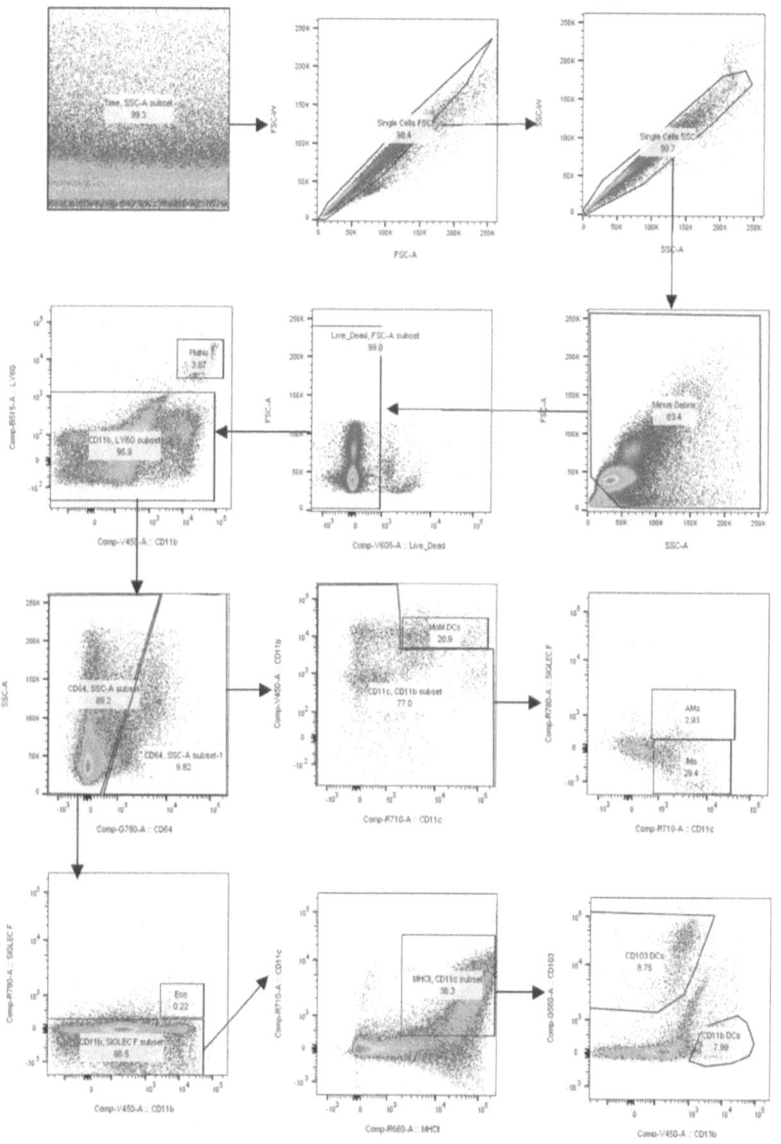

115